CLINICAL MANUAL

for

LARYNGECTOMY

and

HEAD/NECK CANCER

REHABILITATION

Second Edition

D0142503

Clinical Competence Series

Series Editor
Robert T. Wertz, Ph.D.

Clinical Manual for Laryngectomy and Head/Neck Cancer Rehabilitation, Second Edition
Janina K. Casper, Ph.D., and Raymond H. Colton, Ph.D.

Assessment and Intervention Resource for Hispanic Children
Hortencia Kayser, Ph.D.

Approaches to the Treatment of Aphasia
By Nancy Helm-Estabrooks, Sc.D., and Audrey L. Holland, Ph.D.

Developmental Reading Disabilities
Candace L. Goldsworthy, Ph.D.

Effects of Drugs on Communication Disorders
Deanie Vogel, Ph.D., and John E. Carter, M.D.

Manual of Articulation and Phonological Disorders
Ken M. Bleile, Ph.D.

Manual of Assessment and Intervention in Pediatric Bilingual Populations
Hortencia Kayser, Ph.D.

Manual of Voice Treatment: Pediatrics Through Geriatrics
Moya Andrews, Ed.D.

Prosody Management of Communication Disorders
Patricia M. Hargrove, Ph.D., and Nancy S. McGarr, Ph.D.

Right Hemisphere Communication Disorders: Theory and Management
Connie A. Tompkins, Ph.D., CCC-SLP

Sourcebook for Medical Speech Pathology
Lee Ann C. Golper, Ph.D., CCC-SLP

Videoendoscopy: From Velopharynx to Larynx
Michael P. Karnell, Ph.D.

CLINICAL MANUAL
for
LARYNGECTOMY
and
HEAD/NECK CANCER
REHABILITATION

Second Edition

Janina K. Casper, Ph.D.
Associate Professor
Raymond H. Colton, Ph.D.
Professor

Department of Otolaryngology and Communication Sciences
SUNY Health Science Center
Syracuse, New York

With contributions from

Carla DeLassus Gress, Sc.D.
Voice Center
University of California-San Franciscso

SINGULAR PUBLISHING GROUP, INC.
SAN DIEGO · LONDON

Notice: The indications, procedures, drug dosages, and diagnosis and remediation protocols in this book have been recommended in the clinical literature and conform to the practices of the general medical and health services communities. All procedures put forth in this book should be performed only by trained, licensed practitioners. The diagnostic and remediation protocols and the medications described do not necessarily have specific approval by the Food And Drug Administration for use in the disorders and/or diseases and dosages for which they are recommended. Because standards of practice and usage change, it is the responsibility of practitioners to keep abreast of revised recommendations, dosages, and procedures.

Singular Publishing Group, Inc.
401 West A Street, Suite 325
San Diego, California 92101-7904

Singular Publishing Ltd.
19 Compton Terrace
London N1 2UN, UK

© 1998 by Singular Publishing Group, Inc.

Singular Publishing Group, Inc., publishes textbooks, clinical manuals, clinical reference books, journals, videos, and multimedia materials on speech-language pathology, audiology, otorhinolaryngology, special education, early childhood, aging, occupational therapy, physical therapy, rehabilitation, counseling, mental health, and voice. For your convenience, our entire catalog can be accessed on our website at **http//www.singpub.com**. Our mission to provide you with materials to meet the daily challenges of the everchanging health care/educational environment will remain on course if we are in touch with you. In that spirit, we welcome your feedback on our products. Please telephone (**1-800-521-8545**), fax (**1-800-774-8398**), or e-mail (**singpub@mail.cerfnet.com**) your comments and requests to us.

Typeset in 10/12 Times by So Cal Graphics
Printed in the United States of America by McNaughton & Gunn

All rights, including that of translation, reserved. No part of this publication may be reproduced, stored in a retrieval system, or transmitted in any form or by any means, electronic, mechanical, recording, or otherwise, without the prior written permission of the publisher.

Library of Congress Cataloging-in-Publication Data
Casper, Janina K.
    Clinical manual for laryngectomy and head/neck cancer rehabilitation /
Janina K. Casper and Raymond H. Colton; with contributions from
Carla DeLassus Gress. — 2nd ed.
       p.   cm. — (Clinical competence series)
    Includes bibliographical references and index.
    ISBN 1-56593-959-X (spiral: alk. paper)
    1. Head—Cancer—Patients—Rehabilitation.   2. Neck—Cancer
—Patients—Rehabilitation.   3. Laryngectomees—Rehabilitation.
I. Colton, Raymond H.   II. Gress, Carla DeLassus.   III. Title.   IV. Series.
    [DNLM: 1. Laryngectomy—Rehabilitation. 2. Speech, Alaryngeal.
3. Head and Neck Neoplasms—Rehabilitation.   WV 540 C342c 1998]
RC280.H4C38 1998
616.99'42203 — dc21
DNLM/DLC
for Library of Congress   98-17724

CONTENTS

FOREWORD

com•pe•tence (kom´ pə təns) n. The state or quality of being properly or well qualified; capable.

Clinicians crave competence. They pursue it through education and experience, through emulation and innovation. Some are more successful than others in attaining what they seek. Much of being competent is being current. This book, *Clinical Manual for Laryngectomy and Head/Neck Cancer Rehabilitation,* by Drs. Janina K. Casper and Raymond H. Colton, with contributions by Dr. Carla DeLassus Gress, is a second edition. It makes the wealth of information in the first edition current. The contents—Medical/Surgical Examination, Diagnosis, and Treatment; Total Rehabilitation of the Laryngectomee; Alaryngeal Speech; Teaching Alaryngeal Speech; Tracheoesophageal Speech; Characteristics of Alaryngeal and Glossectomy Speech; Oral Cavity Cancer Rehabilitation—cover the ever increasing complexity and technological advances in managing people who suffer communication deficits subsequent to head and neck cancer. The authors wear several hats—teachers; investigators; and, most of all, clinicians. Because they have "been there," they lessen the trepidation associated with seemingly invasive procedures for those of us who have not. Step-by-step explanations of methods prevent us from getting lost. Solutions to combat problems that may arise in restoring communication are offered and generate a sense of security. Certainly, these competent clinicians have provided the information that makes them that way. Our attention to what they present indicates our competence and our efforts to improve it, because competent clinicians seek competence as much for what it demands as for what it promises.

Robert T. Wertz, Ph.D.
Series Editor

PREFACE

Numerous books on voice disorders include a chapter on rehabilitation of patients who have undergone surgical excision of the larynx. It was our feeling, however, that a more detailed, clinically oriented book addressing the full scope of rehabilitation of the patient with head/neck cancer was warranted. In our concept, this includes current approaches to the rehabilitation of the laryngectomized as well as those whose cancer resulted in removal of structures in the oral and/or pharyngeal cavities. Clearly, all of these surgeries have serious consequences for communication and often deglutition. The speech-language pathologist is a primary participant in the rehabilitation process of such patients and must have a clear understanding of the problem.

Although highly clinical in its approach, this book stresses the need for fundamental information about the anatomy of the structures, the nature of their surgical alteration, and the effects on function. Furthermore, information and understanding of the acoustic characteristics of the various modes of speech can guide the clinician in setting appropriate goals. The human side, that is, the recognition of the effects on the person of these various surgical procedures is a constant theme of the book.

The nature of a clinical manual requires that specific procedures be spelled out step-by-step. It is not our intent to have this manual used as a cookbook in the absence of appropriate training and competency. It is our hope that the book will be a significant contribution to the training of speech-language pathologists and will be used throughout the treatment of individuals whose cancer has affected their communication or swallowing ability. We hope this manual will be used selectively to assist the clinician in developing treatment plans appropriate for the needs of each patient.

This second edition is much enhanced by the contributions of Carla DeLassus Gress, Sc.D. Dr. Gress is the author of Chapter 6, which deals with surgical prosthetic voice restoration (tracheoesophageal puncture [TEP]) and tracheoesophageal speech. This material represents current knowledge and state-of-the-art practices. Additional contributions by Dr. Gress are embedded in changes that have been made throughout the book.

Revisions have been made in all chapters in order to update information. There are significant changes in the sections dealing with demographic data and those having to do with electronic speech aids. Although some changes in surgical procedures and techniques have appeared in the literature since the first edition, there are few new, widely practiced approaches in the surgical treatment of head and neck cancers that are appropriate for inclusion in this manual. Nevertheless, some changes have been made, and the illustrations throughout the chapters are from a different source and provide improved clarity.

Chapter 1 presents a general introduction and overview of the diagnosis and treatment of head and neck cancer, its impact on the individual and the family, and demographic data. Chapter 2 reviews some of the procedures used in the examination of the larynx and the basic acoustic and physiologic characteristics of the voice and their measurement. Differential diagnosis and surgical and nonsurgical treatment of carcinoma are presented. Concepts involved in the total rehabilitation of the laryngectomee are explored in Chapter 3. A team approach is stressed, and the roles of the various team members are presented. Consideration is given as well to the needs of the patient, the family, and caregivers. Chapter 4 discusses the various speech modes in some detail, providing descriptions, advantages, disadvantages, and indications for their choice. Chapter 5 presents the basic concepts for the rehabilitation of alaryngeal speech including specific and detailed instructions for teaching mechanical and esophageal speech. Chapter 6 is devoted entirely to the TEP and includes sections on patient selection criteria, insufflation testing, fitting the prosthesis, instruction in voice production, use and care of the prosthesis, the tracheostoma valve, and problems and their solutions. The acoustic, physiological, and perceptual characteristics of alaryngeal speech as well as characteristics of the speech of patients who have had a partial or total glossectomy are described in Chapter 7. Chapter 8 discusses the rehabilitation needs of patients whose head/neck cancer resulted in a loss of parts of the oral or pharyngeal cavities, especially the tongue.

The appendixes have undergone extensive revision and expansion. Appendix A contains a variety of valuable patient education materials that can be copied or adapted for use. Appendix B provides specific guidance in the procedure for videoendoscopic verification of placement of the tracheoesophageal prosthesis and a complete and easy to follow problem-solving guide. Appendix C provides a list of agencies that may be sources of help to the laryngectomee, his or her family and caregivers, and the medical treatment team. Appendix D is a list of suppliers and manufacturers of speech aids, prostheses, amplifiers, and other equipment needed by head and neck cancer patients. A list of materials that can be included in a kit of information for the laryngectomee is provided in Appendix E. Appendix F contains a sample Case History and Assessment form plus a Functional

Communication Rating form that can be used pre- and posttherapy to track outcome from the patient's and the clinician's ratings. And finally, Appendix G is a listing of various Internet sites that should prove valuable for those who work with these challenging problems and desire to stay abreast of new developments as they emerge.

ACKNOWLEDGMENTS

We wish to acknowledge the assistance of Chung Chung, M.D., Richard E. Kelley, M.D., and James Frieje, M.D., all of the SUNY Health Science Center in Syracuse for their input on the current treatment of cancer using radiation oncology and the surgical treatment of head and neck cancers. Martha Hefner, Brian Harris, and Lorraine Davis-Bell of the Medical Illustration section of the Department of Educational Communications, SUNY Health Science Center, provided excellent graphics. We thank Bivona Corporation, InHealth Corporation, Siemens Corporation, and Luminaud Inc. for providing the photographs of various products and materials. Finally, we wish to thank our editor, Marie Linvill, for her encouragement and editorial assistance during the writing of the manuscript.

DEDICATION

With gratitude to our patients from whom we never cease to learn and to our colleagues who have devoted so much of their efforts to further our knowledge and skills in the rehabilitation of this population.

CHAPTER

1

Introduction

I. LARYNGECTOMY

A. Laryngectomy Defined

In its broadest sense, laryngectomy is the surgical procedure in which all or part of the larynx is excised. A total laryngectomy indicates the removal of the entire larynx. Removal of half of the larynx (sagittal cut) is a hemilaryngectomy. Partial laryngectomy denotes excision of less than the total structure. Supraglottic laryngectomy refers to excision of laryngeal structures above the level of the true vocal folds. (See Chapter 2, Section C.2 for more detail.) The person who has had a laryngectomy is commonly referred to as a laryngectomized person or a laryngectomee.

B. Why a Laryngectomy?

The primary indication for laryngectomy is the presence of a malignant tumor of a size and in a location in the larynx that requires surgical removal of the structure en bloc. Size, location, invasiveness, and spread of the tumor will determine the extent of the surgical excision required. A laryngectomy may, on rare occasions, be medically indicated for reasons other than malignancy, such as severe laryngeal trauma, a nonfunctional larynx with intractable aspiration, or irreparable supraglottic stenosis.

Laryngeal trauma may be so severe that the larynx is beyond repair. It may result from direct blows to the larynx, gunshot wounds, severe laceration that severs crucial innervating nerves and/or blood vessels, or damage resulting from motor vehicle injury. A nonfunctional larynx places the patient at risk for life-threatening aspiration in the absence of a mechanism to protect the airway. Thus, a total laryngectomy may be required.

C. Impact on Communication

1. Any laryngectomy, partial or total, will have an effect on voice.

2. A **partial laryngectomy** conserves sufficient laryngeal structure and function to permit audible voice production utilizing pulmonary airflow. The voice quality may be hoarse, breathy, and altered in fundamental frequency and other acoustic parameters.

3. A **total laryngectomy** will render the person at least temporarily voiceless. Although alternative modes of "voicing" are available, they require some form of learning and may depend on the use of an assistive or prosthetic device (see Chapter 4). The resulting voice quality will depend on the mode of voicing used. Until an alternative mode of voicing is established, the person is totally dependent on writing, gesture, or mouthing words to communicate. These latter modes of communication are limited, slow, and often frustrating.

D. Psychological Impact

There are various stages through which a person passes after a laryngectomy, and the primacy of the psychological impact changes and reflects that progression.

1. Preoperative stage. The primary impact during this stage is the knowledge of having cancer. This period is marked by concern about the diagnosis, the surgery, and survival. Secondary concerns at this stage include the obvious sequelae of the surgery, for example, body image, communication, and lifestyle changes.

2. **Early postoperative stage.** Having survived the surgery, primary concern shifts to recovery. The person must adjust to anatomic and body image changes, learn to care for and manage the stoma and various pieces of necessary equipment, and communicate without voice. As the time for discharge from the hospital approaches, feelings of insecurity and fear about the ability to manage physical needs become paramount.

3. **Postdischarge stage.** The long-term effects of the laryngectomy begin to come into sharper focus at this stage. Unless the person has had a primary tracheoesophageal puncture at the time of laryngectomy, concerns about communication may loom larger. Adjustment to all the changes becomes the primary concern as the person resumes aspects of daily life, family life, and social relationships. The nagging fear of recurrence of the cancer may be relegated to the "back burner," but it never totally dissipates. Some patients must undergo radiation therapy, other treatment, or further surgery after the laryngectomy. This creates a new set of concerns and fears, which compound the recovery process.

E. Impact on the Family

Family members experience many of the concerns discussed for the laryngectomized person, but from a different perspective.

1. Initially, there is shock and fear—fear of cancer, fear of the surgery, and fear of the uncertainties of the future.

2. This is followed by the reality of the physical changes that are so apparent and, in the early postsurgical days, can be unpleasant. Although the patient is aware of the changes, the family members see those changes all of the time that they are in the individual's presence. They cannot be avoided. Obvious physical reactions, such as facial grimaces, aversion of gaze, refusal to make eye contact, and crying have a direct impact on the patient. The inability to communicate tends to make everyone uncomfortable. It is especially difficult for young children to see a parent who is physically changed and who is unable to speak.

3. Many frustrations and difficult times follow when the individual returns home but cannot fully resume the role formerly played in the family. There is a tendency for family members to view the individual as diminished in all ways. All family members must adjust to a new form of communication, which may range

from very easy to understand to almost impossible. The frustration on all sides can be enormous. Families can benefit a great deal from contact with others who have been through the experience and from counselors who are sensitive to the issues.

F. Economic Impact

The economic impact of a laryngectomy can be multifocal.

1. **Medical/surgical costs.** A major surgical procedure carries a very high price tag. Even for those patients with adequate insurance coverage, the process of managing the bills and understanding insurance company statements can be extremely difficult and intimidating. A large percentage of patients will have Medicare coverage that may be inadequate. They may be required to pay a percentage of the costs, which can be an onerous burden. Others may have no insurance coverage and be unable to assume the costs personally.

2. **Income.** A fairly lengthy period of sick leave may be required for employed persons. Policies of employers vary in their coverage for such leave. Some persons may be unable to return to their presurgical jobs. These are important concerns for persons whose income is essential for the survival of the family and its life-style.

3. **Rehabilitation.** There are costs associated with rehabilitation, including those for alaryngeal speech training, purchase of assistive or prosthetic devices, and transportation to and parking at the location where rehabilitation is provided. Rehabilitation may be a covered service through various third party payors, but for the person who is uninsured or insufficiently insured, the costs may be greater than the individual is able to absorb.

II. NEED FOR EARLY AND ONGOING LARYNGECTOMEE REHABILITATION

As the preceding sections demonstrate, there are numerous problems and adjustments that the person faced with the diagnosis of laryngeal cancer encounters. "Effective rehabilitation depends on appropriate early treatment decisions" (Myers, Barofsky, & Yates, 1986). The help of professionals from various disciplines is needed to assist the patient. Some of these professionals are involved in all stages, from diagnosis through rehabilitation. Others may play a more limited role. (See Chapter 3 for a detailed description of the rehabilitation team.)

A. Psychosocial

The patient's ability to accept the diagnosis and the recommended course of treatment is of primary importance from the moment of diagnosis. The patient who has difficulty with this may reject treatment and be lost to follow-up, thereby risking many years of life. It is critical that these patients be followed with sensitivity and care and be provided with the necessary support services early in the process. During both the early postoperative period and the postdischarge stage, patients may experience depression. This may be expressed in various forms, must be recognized, and assistance provided. Depression can compromise the patient's recovery, retard physical healing, and be a hindrance to initiating alaryngeal communication training.

B. Swallowing

Some patients may encounter swallowing difficulty when nasal tube feedings are stopped. This is the case when the patient has had a subtotal laryngectomy procedure or extensive surgery with lingual resection and/or hypopharyngeal or esophageal reconstruction. (See Chapters 3 and 7 for more details of swallowing rehabilitation.)

1. Almost all persons who undergo supraglottic laryngectomy experience swallowing problems in the early postoperative period. It is critical that the person master the ability to swallow without aspiration, a problem that can be life threatening. The person who continues to have significant aspiration may eventually face a total laryngectomy.

2. Loss of significant portions of the tongue or restriction in its movement will make it difficult to propel the bolus in preparation for swallowing. Once again, early assistance with this problem is indicated.

3. The esophageal lumen may be constricted in some persons, particularly if they have required extensive pharyngeal or esophageal reconstruction. This constriction hinders the passage of food, and repeated esophageal dilatations may be required. Adjusted eating and swallowing habits must be learned.

C. Speech

Loss of the ability to produce voice for speech, laughter, and crying is the single most profound handicap that results from laryngectomy. Writing or shaping words without sound are usually unsatisfactory methods of communication. The absence of the ability to express oneself can cause or contribute to a sense of isolation and depression. It is urgent that the person be made aware of the available options for alaryngeal speech and of the time course for the acquisition or initiation of these options soon after the diagnosis is made. At the earliest postoperative time possible, the patient should be provided with a means of communication. (See Chapter 4 for a detailed discussion of alaryngeal speech options.)

III. ETIOLOGY OF LARYNGECTOMY: INCIDENCE, PREVALENCE, AND SURVIVAL

Data about incidence, prevalence, survival, and risk for laryngeal cancer are available from sources such as the National Cancer Institute and the National American Cancer Society (see Appendix G for internet sites) and are published in the journal *CA—A Cancer Journal for Clinicians*. Statistics are gathered annually, and those provided here were gathered or estimated for the years cited.

A. Laryngeal Carcinoma

1. Etiology

a. Smoking of cigarettes, pipes, or cigars is a significant etiological factor in the development of laryngeal cancer in men and women. It is directly related to measures of use such as amount and duration of the smoking habit. Ten years after cessation of smoking, mortality risks are the same as those for nonsmokers. Smokers of filtered cigarettes have a slightly reduced level of risk than those who smoke unfiltered cigarettes.

b. There appears to be a synergistic effect between smoking and alcohol intake that increases the level of risk for laryngeal cancer. For a heavy drinker who smokes an average of 35 cigarettes per day, there is a 22.1% risk of developing laryngeal cancer. The relative risk of developing laryngeal cancer is increased by 50% more than would be predicted by the simple additive effect when tobacco and alcohol abuse are combined.

c. The "typical" person diagnosed with laryngeal cancer is a 60-year-old man who is a heavy smoker with moderate to heavy alcohol intake. However, the incidence of this disease in women has been rising in recent years.

d. There is a recognized interaction between smoking and occupational exposure to various chemicals and other substances. One of the best documented interactions related to the development of laryngeal cancer is the synergistic effect of smoking and asbestos exposure. "Both smoke and some industrial pollutants contain substances capable of initiating and promoting cancer. There is, therefore, an ample biologic basis for suspecting that important interactive effects between some work place pollutants and tobacco smoke exist" (U.S. Department of Health and Human Services, 1986).

e. Although we are aware of families in whom more than a single member has had laryngeal cancer, there is as yet no well documented genetic link to development of cancer of the larynx. Increased familial incidence is recognized.

f. Research continues to explore the role of diet in the development of all cancers. It is estimated that one third of the 500,000 yearly deaths from cancer in the United States are due to dietary factors. We are not aware of any studies that have specifically targeted laryngeal cancer. However, the Advisory Committee on Diet, Nutrition, and Cancer Prevention of the American Cancer Society has provided guidelines for reducing the risk of cancer with healthy food choices and physical activity. The main recommendations include: (1) stay within a healthy weight range; (2) engage in at least 30 minutes of moderate physical activity per day; (3) reduce saturated fat intake; (4) eat mostly food from plant sources (i.e., fruits, vegetables, grains, beans).

g. Radiation-induced laryngeal tumors, although uncommon, have been reported.

2. Demographics

a. Cancer is the second leading cause of death in the United States following heart disease. Laryngeal cancer accounts for less than 1% of all cancers and about 6% of all cancers of the respiratory system.

b. Data reported in *CA—A Cancer Journal for Clinicians* estimated about 9,000 new cases of laryngeal cancer in males in the United States and 2,100 new cases in females for the year 1998. Estimated numbers of deaths from laryngeal cancer in 1998 are given as 3,400 males and 900 females. The male to female ratio is about 5:1 for both blacks and whites. Although the incidence of laryngeal cancer has historically been much greater for males than females, the ratio has been changing as increased numbers of women are diagnosed with laryngeal cancer.

c. According to the Surveillance, Epidemiology, and End Results (SEER) study the incidence of laryngeal cancer showed a slight decrease for whites of both sexes for the years 1990–1994 as compared to the mid-1980s. Blacks showed a slight increase over the same time period. Mortality decreased slightly for whites of both sexes but increased slightly for blacks of both sexes.

d. The average annual incidence of laryngeal cancer per 100,000 population for the years 1974–1994 is reported by the National Cancer Institute SEER program. The statistics by age and sex are presented in Table 1–1. It is clear that incidence rates rise sharply in the fifth, sixth, and first half of the seventh decades of life. Incidence begins to decline in the last half of the seventh decade. The greater incidence among blacks, both male and female, compared to whites, is also apparent.

e. There is some evidence to suggest that squamous cell cancer in different parts of the larynx may have different etiological

Table 1–1. Average annual laryngeal cancer incidence rates per 100,000 population by age, sex, and race.

Race/Sex	Age Group							
	45–49	*50–54*	*55–59*	*60–64*	*65–69*	*70–74*	*75–79*	*80–84*
White male	5.6	12.6	20.4	29.7	41.3	39.6	44.5	35.6
White female	1.3	2.9	5.6	6.7	8.6	6.7	7.0	4.4
Black male	16.3	25.1	42.6	66.5	62.3	67.1	44.6	50.6
Black female	2.5	8.4	9.6	7.0	15.0	8.9	6.9	9.8

Source: Adapted from Ries, L.A.G., Kosch, P.C., Hankey, B.F., Miller, C.J., & Harras, A. *SEER Cancer Statistics Review, 1973–94.* (1997). Bethesda, MD: National Cancer Institute. NIH Pub. No. 97-2789.

influences, and thus differ in incidence as well. Yang, Thomas, Daling, and Davis (1989) reported a substantially higher male to female ratio for cancers in the glottic region than in other subsites, and a rapid increase in these ratios as a function of age. These findings suggest that hormonal or other sex-related factors may be involved etiologically and not solely smoking and drinking.

f. Five-year relative survival rates by race, reported by Ries et al. (1997), demonstrate not only a greater percentage of survival in whites than blacks, but also show an increase in the percentage of survival since 1974 for whites and a decrease for blacks (Figure 1–1). These are shown in Table 1–2. No explanation for this decrease is provided. However, it is known that diagnosis of cancer in its early localized stage, when chances for cure are best, occurs less often in blacks (33%) than in whites (39%). Thus, if the condition is in a more advanced stage at diagnosis for blacks, the outcome of treatment would be less favorable.

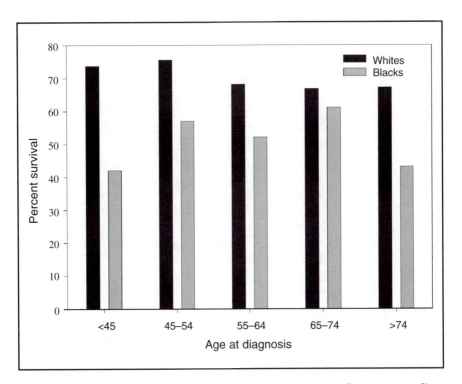

Figure 1–1. Five-year survival rate for blacks and whites according to age at diagnosis. (Data from Reis et al., 1997.)

Table 1–2. Five-year relative survival rates for patients with laryngeal cancer.

Years	% Whites	% Blacks
1974–76	66.5	58.3
1977–79	68.2	56.0
1980–82	69.3	58.5
1983–85	69.3	55.5
1986–93	69.1	54.2

Source: Adapted from Ries, L.A.G., Kosch, P.C., Hankey, B.F., Miller, C.J., & Harras, A. *SEER Cancer Statistics Review, 1973–94.* (1997). Bethesda, MD: National Cancer Institute. NIH Pub. No. 97-2789.

B. Nonfunctional Larynx

1. Etiology

a. A laryngectomy may become necessary when the larynx is nonfunctional. The loss of the protective function of the larynx in guarding the airway presents a major threat to life. Reasons for a nonfunctional larynx may include:

(1) A failed subtotal laryngectomy procedure. If a subtotal laryngectomy procedure results in a nonfunctional larynx, a complete laryngectomy may be indicated.

(2) Traumatic injury so severe that laryngeal reconstruction is impossible.

(3) Severe supraglottic stenosis may require that a supraglottic laryngectomy be performed.

(4) Loss of central nervous system control of laryngeal function such as might occur following a brain stem stroke.

(5) Radiation chondritis (inflammation) may be so severe as to warrant total laryngectomy.

2. Demographics

a. There are no data available for nonfunctional larynx patients as a group. Instances of laryngectomy being performed for the problems described above but in the absence of cancer, are known; however, they are rare.

CHAPTER

2

Medical/Surgical Examination, Diagnosis, and Treatment

Proper medical care requires a thorough examination prior to diagnosis or initiation of treatment. Otolaryngologists use a variety of procedures to examine the larynx. Most are visual and allow the examiner to view laryngeal structures without anesthesia or surgical procedures. Others are indirect measures that provide evaluation of voice function. A common symptom of laryngeal cancer is hoarseness, thus it is important to note the disturbances of phonatory function. Furthermore, it is necessary to understand those acoustic parameters that are altered in alaryngeal speech. Measurement of these provides important information about the nature and adequacy of various modes of alaryngeal speech.

I. EXAMINATION PROCEDURES

A. Indirect Mirror Examination

The simplest, initial examination is conducted by placing an angled mirror in the back of the mouth behind the faucial pillars while directing a beam of light via a head mirror to illuminate the vocal folds and other structures of the larynx. No anesthesia is needed, and the examination technique can be learned quickly and requires a minimum of technical knowledge. Interpretation of the results, however, requires complete knowledge of laryngeal anatomy, physiology, and pathology. The image may be viewed only briefly, because the patient can only sustain a sound for a short time period. Some patients have a sensitive gag reflex that may be triggered with this procedure. There is usually no recorded documentation of the indirect mirror examination, and phonation is limited to a sustained vowel /i/. This sound is used because it is a high front vowel that brings the epiglottis forward and dilates the lower pharynx and laryngeal vestibule, thereby permitting optimal visualization of the vocal folds.

B. Fiberoptic Examination

1. The Fiberscope

The fiberoptic endoscope is an instrument made up of a bundle of fibers, some of which carry light down to the larynx while other fibers pass the image up to the eyepiece. The image can be seen by the examiner through an eyepiece, or the endoscope can be coupled to a video camera making it possible to view the image on a monitor and videotape the examination. The tape provides a record for review of the examination, documentation of findings, and a means to assess changes resulting from treatment. Endoscopes can be of the rigid or the flexible type. The rigid scope is angled at the posterior end so that when positioned through the mouth into the oropharynx a view of the vocal folds can be obtained. This scope has some of the same limitations as the mirror examination (e.g., occasional difficulty in visualizing the laryngeal inlet and the folds, may evoke gag reflex, limits the utterance to sustained vowel), but it provides an enhanced image. When equipped with videotaping capability, the image on the monitor is enlarged, can be reviewed, and provides a documented record. The flexible fiberoptic endoscope is passed through one of patient's nares and positioned above the entrance to the larynx and, if possible, directly over the vocal folds (Figure 2–1).

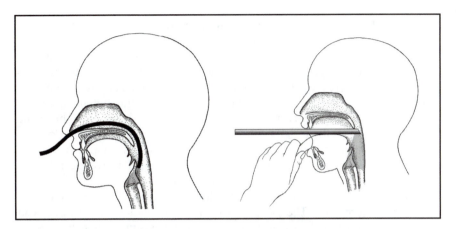

Figure 2–1. Schematic of an examination of the larynx using a rigid endoscope (right panel) or a flexible laryngoscope (left panel).

It may be helpful, but not always necessary, to administer some topical anesthetic (Hurricaine, Xylocaine, Pontocaine, etc.) prior to insertion of the endoscope to reduce the sensitivity felt by some patients. Because the fiberscope is not placed through the mouth, gagging is greatly reduced. The light source is continuous.

2. Speech Tasks

With the flexible endoscope in place, the patient is free to perform a variety of speech tasks, including words and sentences. A typical protocol might include visualization of the larynx at rest, during the production of sustained vowels at various pitch levels, while saying sentences and perhaps during whistling. The latter is a good maneuver to assess the movement of the arytenoids and vocal folds during abduction/adduction.

C. Stroboscopy

Stroboscopy permits direct visualization of the vibration of the vocal folds, although the image obtained is, in reality, an illusion. Stroboscopy is based on the principle that the human eye retains a visual image for a small but finite period of time, usually 0.2 seconds. By flashing an interrupted light at the proper rate, an illusion of slow motion can be obtained of a system that is, in reality, vibrating very rapidly.

1. To perform a **stroboscopic examination of the vocal folds**, a rigid endoscope is positioned far back in the oropharynx (or a flexible endoscope is passed through the nose) to provide a view of the larynx. A microphone is held to the side of the neck to record the acoustic output of the vocal folds. The stroboscope unit extracts the fundamental frequency from this output, which, in turn, controls the flashing rate of the stroboscopic light. If the strobe light flashes at the same rate as the fundamental frequency of the vocal folds, the image will be static, or if the signal is very aperiodic, some movement may be revealed. However, if the rate of the strobe light flash is slightly different from the fundamental frequency of the vocal folds, an illusion of slow motion is obtained. The patient must produce a sustained vowel but can vary fundamental frequency and/or intensity of phonation.

2. **Stroboscopy has contributed much to our understanding of vocal fold vibration in health and disease**. It is valuable for diagnosing polyps, nodules, cysts, edema, and scarring. It can be used to differentiate functional problems from those caused by structural abnormalities or disease. Woo, Colton, Casper, and Brewer (1991) reported that, of 195 patients, the diagnoses of 10% were changed as a result of stroboscopic examination. Included in this sample were 3 patients with laryngeal cancer whose treatment was changed from hemilaryngectomy to laser cordectomy based on the improved ability to differentiate superficial from deeply invasive disease.

3. The **stroboscopic image provides information** about the symmetry and movement of the vocal folds, the regularity of their motion, the degree of glottal closure, the degree of horizontal excursion of the vocal folds, the presence of nonvibrating segments, and information about the effect of lesions on vocal fold vibratory function. Hirano and Bless (1993) have described the principles of stroboscopy and the various observations and judgments that can be made from the stroboscopic image. It is clear, however, that complete and accurate understanding of vibratory motion requires a thorough understanding of the anatomy and physiology of phonation as well as adequate training in the visualization and interpretation of stroboscopic images.

D. Other Procedures

1. Acoustic analysis

a. **Fundamental Frequency (F_0) of phonation reflects the vibrating rate of the vocal folds**. The unit of measurement is Hertz (Hz). It can be measured during sustained phonation or during connected speech. The techniques for measuring fundamental frequency in these two conditions may be different, and the instrumentation available ranges from simple to complex. The simplest utterance to measure is the sustained vowel. The F_0 of connected utterances requires more sophisticated instrumentation or specialized computer programs.

b. **Fundamental Frequency Variation reflects the variation in the vibrating rate of the vocal folds;** a variation that may be affected by disease or lesions of the vocal folds. Two kinds of variability can be measured: short term (*perturbation*) and long term (*pitch sigma*). Pertubation refers to the rapid variations of fundamental frequency and is thought to reflect instabilities in the vocal folds or their neural control. It is correlated with the perception of hoarseness. Perturbation is computed by subtracting successive periods and averaging differences over the number of cycles. It is usually expressed in a ratio, although absolute measures of time may be used. Pitch sigma is the standard deviation of fundamental frequency and reflects, in addition to perturbation, the longer time variation of F_0 that may reflect linguistic, semantic, or psychological demands. It is reported in Hz or in seimtones FL.

c. **Phonational Range is the largest range of F_0s a patient can produce.** It is obtained by finding the lowest and highest frequencies the patient can sustain for a short period of time, usually 1 second without regard to voice intensity or quality. Although it may be expressed in Hz, it is more often reported in terms of semitones Frequency Level (FL).

d. **Vocal Intensity is a reflection of the acoustic power produced by the vibrating vocal folds** as well as the effects of the vocal tract or sound resonator. Vocal intensity at the level of the vocal folds is dependent on the effectiveness of the vocal folds in achieving glottal closure, which allows a buildup of air pressure below the vocal folds. Vocal intensity can be measured using a microphone together with a sound level meter, specialized sound level recorders, or computer-based systems. Intensity is expressed in decibels (dB). It can be measured using sustained vowels or connected speech. For measurement of a sustained vowel, a simple (and in some cases inexpensive) sound level meter can be used. Connected speech requires more complex measurement procedures.

e. **Variation of Vocal Intensity**, like F_0, may be measured between successive cycles of phonation (*shimmer*) or a much larger number of cycles (*standard deviation*). Shimmer, like perturbation, reflects the stability of the vocal folds and is correlated with hoarseness. The amplitude of each vibratory cycle is subtracted from the previous one, averaged over all such differences, and expressed in dB of change. Standard deviation of vocal intensity reflects variation occurring over a longer time period.

f. **Dynamic Range is the range of intensities a person can produce from the softest to the loudest.** The difference between the two is the dynamic range (in dB). Dynamic range is a reflection of the person's phonatory abilities and should increase as more efficient phonation is achieved.

g. **Acoustic Spectrum results from an analysis of the amplitudes of the component frequencies of a tone.** It is the major acoustic correlate of voice quality. It is expressed in a variety of ways, but the most common are spectrograms, spectral plots, and long-term average spectrum.

   (1) **Spectrograms** portray frequency and intensity information as a function of time. They have been used for the analysis of speech production as well as dynamic acoustic events in other disciplines. In most cases, spectrograms can illustrate the varied frequency characteristics of different acoustic events. A spectrogram can be made with specialized instruments (Kay Elemetrics Corporation Sona-graph) or with computer-based software and hardware (CSpeech, CSL, EZVoice, MacSpeech Lab, etc.).

   (2) **A spectral plot** is a snapshot of the frequencies present in a tone at a specific moment in time. Frequency spectrum is usually plotted by locating the frequencies along the horizontal axis and the intensity of each frequency along the vertical axis.

   (3) **Long-term average spectrum (LTAS)** refers to a procedure where successive spectra of an utterance are computed and averaged together to provide an estimate of the typical or average spectrum of the utterance. It can be an important technique for the analysis of abnormal voice since it reflects the overall spectral characteristics of the voice rather than any short-term spectrum that might be associated with a specific vowel or consonant.

2. Vibratory Analysis

a. Inverse Filtered Airflow is a procedure where the effects of the oral resonances are removed from the orally emitted waveform leaving an estimate of the airflow pattern through the vocal folds. It requires an airflow system capable of responding to frequencies to about 1200 Hz and adjustable inverse filters to remove the resonances. This device is available from a commercial source (Glottal Enterprises) and has a moderate cost. It has been used clinically to analyze the airflow characteristics of a variety of voice problems. In addition to measuring F_0, the peak and leakage airflow through the glottis, Open Quotient (percentage of time the vocal folds are open divided by the total time of a cycle), and Speed Quotient (time it takes for the vocal folds to open divided by the time it takes for them to close) can be measured.

b. Electroglottography is an indirect method for the measurement of vocal fold opening and closing. The electroglottograph (EGG) passes a high frequency current through the neck and measures the impedance of the tissues and structures in the neck to this current flow. A small portion of the total impedance across the neck is due to the vibrating vocal folds. This small fraction is detected by the device, amplified, and can be displayed on an oscilloscope or computer screen (if appropriate hardware and software are used). With the aid of an appropriate model of vocal fold vibration, the opening, closing, and closed portions can be identified. An Abduction Quotient (roughly the percentage of the time the vocal folds are open divided by the total time of the vocal fold cycle) and closing times of the vocal folds may be determined from the output of an EGG.

c. Photoglottography is a technique where light is passed through the vocal folds and detected using a light meter or photocell. The amount of light is an approximate indication of the area of opening of the vocal folds. From these data, measurements of F_0, Open Quotient, and Speed Quotient can be made.

E.   Direct Laryngoscopy with Biopsy

1. Direct laryngoscopy is a procedure usually requiring hospitalization. It is sometimes necessary when the physician suspects a tumor or other abnormal tissue growth. A biopsy involves obtaining a small sample of the suspected tissue and submitting it to analysis by a pathologist.

2. With the patient under general anesthesia, **a laryngoscope is inserted in the mouth and pharynx allowing direct visualization of the larynx and vocal folds**. This procedure provides optimum views of the larynx at rest and allows the use of instruments for manipulating structures or excising biopsy tissue. A long, fine pair of scissors or forceps is passed through the tube and positioned over the suspected tissue area. A small sample is taken and sent to the pathology lab for analysis. When it is important to determine the histology of the tissue, this procedure is essential to confirm a diagnosis, especially when malignancy is suspected.

II. DIFFERENTIAL DIAGNOSIS

A. Cancer Staging

1. Development of Cancer

Cancer rarely appears full-blown in an individual. More often, cancer develops from a single area and expands to include more and more of the area. Eventually, it may metastasize, that is, extend to more remote areas of the body via passage through the blood or lymphatic system. The cancer staging system has been developed and refined over many years in an attempt to define the extent and severity of the cancer and to assist in planning treatment.

2. TNM System

Cancer staging is usually reported using the TNM system (American Joint Committee on Cancer, 1977; see Table 2–1). In this system, the "T" identifies the location of the primary tumor. Thus, a T0 classification indicates no evidence of a tumor, whereas a T4 classification indicates a massive tumor involving the structure of interest (in our case, the larynx). The "N" in the system refers to the involvement of the lymph nodes in the immediate region, in this context, the neck. An Nx means that lymph node involvement cannot be assessed, whereas an N3 refers to massive lymph node involvement. The "M" component of the system indicates the extent of tumor spread or metastasis. Thus, a patient with the classification T3N1M0 has a moderately large

Table 2–1. TNM System for staging of cancer of the larynx.

Primary Tumor (T)	Glottis	Regional Lymph Nodes (N)
TX Primary tumor cannot be assessed T0 No evidence of primary tumor Tis Carcinoma in situ	T1 Tumor limited to the vocal cord(s) (may involve anterior or posterior commissure) with normal mobility T1a Tumor limited to one vocal cord T1b Tumor involves both vocal cords T2 Tumor extends to supraglottis and/or subglottis, and/or with impaired vocal cord mobility T3 Tumor limited to the larynx with vocal cord fixation T4 Tumor invades through the thyroid cartilage and/or to other tissues beyond the larynx (e.g., the trachea, soft tissues of the neck, including thyroid, pharynx)	NX Regional lymph nodes cannot be assessed N0 No regional lymph node metastasis N1 Metastasis in a single ipsilateral lymph node, 3 cm or less in the greatest dimension N2 Metastasis in a single ipsilateral lymph node, more than 3 cm but not more than 6 cm in the greatest dimension, or in multiple ipsilateral lymph nodes, none more than 6 cm in the greatest dimension, or in bilateral or contralateral lymph nodes, none more than 6 cm in the greatest dimension N2a Metastasis in a single ipsilateral lymph node more than 3 cm but not more than 6 cm in the greatest dimension N2b Metastasis in multiple ipsilateral lymph nodes, none more than 6 cm in the greatest dimension N2c Metastasis in bilateral or contralateral lymph nodes, none more than 6 cm in the greatest dimension N3 Metastasis in a lymph node more than 6 cm in the greatest dimension *(continued)*

Table 2–1. *(continued)*

Supraglottis	Subglottis	Distant Metastasis (M)
T1 Tumor limited to one subsite of the supraglottis with normal vocal cord mobility T2 Tumor invades mucosa of more than one adjacent subsite of the supraglottis or glottis or a region outside the supraglottis (e.g., mucosa of base of tongue, vallecula, medial wall of the pyriform sinus) without fixation of the larynx T3 Tumor limited to the larynx with vocal cord fixation and/or invades any of the following: postcricoid area, pre-epiglottic tissues T4 Tumor invades through the thyroid cartilage, and/or extends into soft tissues of the neck, thyroid, and/or esophagus	T1 Tumor limited to the subglottis T2 Tumor extends to the vocal cord(s) with normal or impaired mobility T3 Tumor limited to the larynx with vocal cord fixation T4 Tumor invades through the cricoid or thyroid cartilage and/or extends to other tissues beyond the larynx (e.g., trachea, soft tissues of the neck, including the thyroid, esophagus)	MX Distant metastasis cannot be assessed MO No distant metastasis M1 Distant metastasis

Source: Adapted from American Joint Committee on Cancer. (1997). *Manual for Staging of Cancer* (5th ed.), Philadelphia: Lippincott-Raven.

tumor with some small involvement of the regional nodes but no spread of the tumor. The TNM classification classifies a tumor and assists in choosing the treatment modality most likely to be successful.

B. Types of Laryngeal Cancers and Their Histological Characteristics

There are several types of cancer that can be differentiated by a pathologist based on analysis of the cells present in the biopsy. *Squamous cell carcinoma* is the most common laryngeal type (greater than 95%) which manifests itself as a thickening of the epithelial surface, although exact details will vary according to the site at which it is found. For example, in the glottic area during the early stage, the mucosal surface may show an irregular thickening with a possible whitish, cauliflower appearance. At later stages, it may be seen as an impairment of vocal fold motion. Supraglottic sites may be manifested by a tumor with raised edges and multiple areas of ulceration. Subglottic tumors may be diffuse and appear whitish or reddish in coloration. Histological analysis describes the cellular structure of a lesion as well, moderately, or poorly differentiated. In general, a more differentiated carcinoma is associated with a better prognosis.

A more rare neoplasm is *verrucous carcinoma* which is somewhat hyperkeratotic in appearance, seemingly benign but really malignant. Also rare in the larynx are the *sarcomas* (fibrosarcoma, rhabdomyosarcoma, chondrosarcoma, etc.), *spindle cell carcinoma*, and *adenocarcinoma*. Occasionally, a *metastatic carcinoma* of the larynx may be found with the primary site elsewhere in the body, most frequently the kidneys, prostate, breast, or gastrointestinal tract. Also rare is *oat cell carcinoma*, a neoplasm usually found in the bronchi.

C. Signs and Symptoms of Carcinoma in Head and Neck

1. Symptoms of Carcinoma

The most common symptom (patient complaint) of laryngeal cancer is *hoarseness*. Hoarseness will occur when the true vocal folds are sufficiently involved to disrupt vibratory behavior. It is possible, however, that the carcinoma may be advanced when this symptom occurs, particularly if the primary site is elsewhere in the larynx. For large tumors, *dyspnea* (difficulty breathing) and *stridor* (audible passage of air during breathing) may be present. Glottic tumors may produce both inspiratory and expiratory stridor, whereas supraglottic tumors may be associated with *inspiratory* stridor and subglottic tumors with *expiratory* stridor. *Pain* may occur in patients with hypopharyngeal, epiglottic, or pyriform sinus cancer. *Dysphagia* may occur in cancers of the tongue, supraglottic areas, or pyriform sinus. Other possible symptoms are *coughing* and/or *hemoptysis* (blood expectoration). Other symptoms are weight loss, halitosis, swelling in the neck, and tenderness in the laryngeal area.

2. Signs of Carcinoma

Some signs (observable, measurable manifestations) of laryngeal carcinoma may be noted from a routine neck examination or from examination of the larynx and vocal folds. From the *neck examination*, it is possible to discover: (1) a lump in the neck, (2) tenderness in the laryngeal area, (3) lack of sound (crepitation) on side to side movement of the larynx, (4) fullness in the cricothyroid or thyrohyoid membrane, and/or (5) presence of lumps at the base of the tongue.

3. Examination of the larynx may reveal different clinical signs depending on the location of the tumor. Tumors on the true vocal folds appear as irregular lesions, whitish in appearance, that may range from a very small size to a very large tumor that prevents movement of parts or all of the vocal fold. Supraglottic lesions may manifest themselves as piled-up tissue with ulcerations. Subglottic lesions may appear whitish or reddish, diffuse in appearance, and with some evidence of superficial ulcerations. Carcinoma-in-situ is a localized lesion of the true vocal fold that appears whitish and looks somewhat like hyperkeratosis.

III. TREATMENT

A. Radiation Therapy

1. Rationale

For some kinds of carcinoma, the **primary treatment modality is often radiation therapy** (Figure 2–2). New instrumentation and techniques have greatly increased the effectiveness of radiation therapy thereby leading to increased survival of patients with laryngeal carcinoma. Using a combined treatment approach, along with surgery and/or chemotherapy, radiation therapy has increased the success of surgery. However, radiation therapy cannot be used with every patient, and there are definite indications for its use. All cells will respond to radiation although the more rapidly growing cells will be more affected by the irradiation.

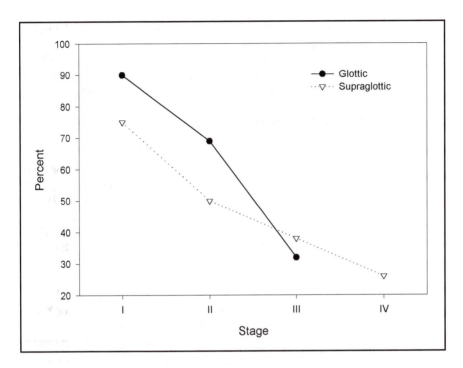

Figure 2–2. Survival percentage with irradiation alone for carcinoma of the supra-glottic and glottis. (Based on data presented by Brady, L. W., & Davis, L. W. [1988]. Treatment of head and neck cancer by radiation therapy. *Seminars in Oncology, 15,* 29–38.)

2. Indications

The primary goals of radiation therapy are to achieve tumor control and to preserve voice. Spector and Ogura (1985) recommended radiation therapy as the primary treatment modality for three kinds of laryngeal tumors: (1) small, superficial tumors of one or both true vocal folds; (2) tumors that involve the free border of the epiglottis and are less than 1 cm in diameter; and (3) tumors in patients who are a poor risk for surgery. Cure rates for irradiated T1 lesions are similar to those achieved with surgery, whereas the control of T2 lesions with radiation alone is slightly less favorable. Some surgeons may use radiation therapy for slightly more extensive lesions.

3. Dosage

The techniques for radiation therapy have evolved over the years as more experience has been gained with this form of treatment.

Currently, megavoltage units are in use, because they are more penetrating, have less scattering, and have a reduced effect on the skin.

The division of the total amount of radiation is important in achieving success in tumor control. Usually, patients with laryngeal cancer are given 6000 cGy in 30 fractions over a period of about 6 weeks. Newer procedures, such as hyper-fractionation, will deliver approximately the same daily dosage but on a twice a day schedule, whereas in some patients, a higher dosage may be used but only within a specified target zone. These newer procedures, most often used for T3 or T4 tumors, have shown promise in reducing or eliminating tumors and yielding greater long-term control of a tumor. More extensive tumors may require more irradiation; a longer time course; and, in some cases, may be combined with chemotherapy.

In some patients, irradiation is used in conjunction with surgery. If radiation is given presurgically, it can result in hardening of the tissues, making surgery more difficult, or it can result in slower or more incomplete wound healing. The preferred approach, when radiation and surgery are combined, is for the surgery to be done first to reduce the risk of morbidity.

4. Morbidity

Patients who undergo radiation therapy may experience changes in swallowing, changes in voice quality, xerostomia with mucositis and reduced salivary flow, and reduction in lingual and mandibular range of motion. Some of these effects may be temporary, and most are treatable to some extent.

B. Surgery

1. Hemilaryngectomy

This procedure is also known as Vertical Partial Laryngectomy.

a. **Anatomic and Physiologic Changes.** With this surgical technique, generally one of the true vocal folds is removed along with the vocal process of the corresponding arytenoid. In some cases, it may be necessary to remove the entire arytenoid. Occasionally, it may be necessary to remove a limited portion of the opposite cord. In addition, the tissue between the vocal folds and the thyroid ala is removed, leaving a large defect. The excised vocal fold area is reconstructed with muscle. Figure 2–3 shows the anatomical changes that may occur after this operation. Physiologically, the major effect is the disruption in voice. The postsurgical voice is often hoarse, very breathy, and weak. There may be some disturbance of swallowing; of short duration for some and longer lasting for others. Patients may need to learn new strategies for producing voice and swallowing.

b. Indications for Use. This procedure is used for primary and recurrent tumors involving the glottis. Extension of the lesion should not be more than 1 cm below the free edges of the vocal fold. The floor of the ventricle may also be involved. The procedure can be very effective in achieving tumor control, even in patients with a more extensive lesion (see Table 2–2).

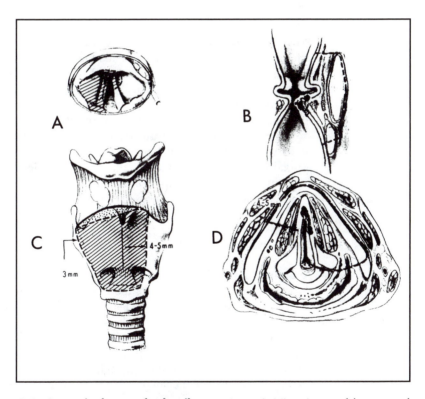

Figure 2–3. Anatomic changes after hemilaryngectomy. A. Mirror image of the extent of the carcinoma with a schematic representation of resected tissue. Note that aryepiglottic folds are not included in the vertical laryngectomy. **B.** Frontal section depicts the depth of the resection to include: the true vocal fold, the false vocal fold and walls of ventricle, the lateral subglottic tissue with cricothyroid membrane and upper one half of cricoid cartilage, and the thyroid ala preserving its outer perichondrium. **C.** Anterior schematic drawing depicting the extent of the thyroid cartilage resected as delineated by the broken line. A modification superiorly is along the solid line. **D.** Cross section depicts extent of resection described previously. (From Loré, J. M. [1988]. *An Atlas of Head and Neck Surgery* [3rd ed.]. Philadelphia: W. B. Saunders Company. Used by permission.)

Table 2–2. Survival rates for hemilaryngectomy.

Tumor Stage	Percent 3-Year NED*
T1	87
T2	82
T3	90

*NED = No evidence of disease

Source: Adapted from Kaiser, T. N., and Spector, G. J., Tumors of the larynx and laryngopharynx. In Ballenger, J. J. (Ed.), Diseases of the nose, throat, ear, head, and neck (14th ed.) (pp. 682–746). Philadelphia: Lea & Febiger.

c. **Pros and Cons.** Hemilaryngectomy can be very effective in achieving tumor control with a limited removal of tissue. The voice, although dysphonic, remains usable. Swallowing problems, when present, tend to be easily handled. Patients do not have side effects associated with irradiation. Hemilaryngectomy may also be used for salvage of radiation failures for small glottic tumors. Reconstruction of the posterior portions of the vocal folds during the procedure avoids a problem with aspiration. The patient may experience airway problems for a short time after the operation. On the negative side, the voice is not as good as that obtained after a course of irradiation alone, which has similar survival rates.

2. **Supraglottic Laryngectomy**

a. **Anatomic and Physiologic Changes.** Supraglottic refers to those laryngeal structures above the level of the glottis. Resection can include removal of the hyoid bone, if it is involved, along with the entire ventricular folds, the epiglottis, and part of the thyroid cartilage (see Figure 2–4). As a result of loss of these structures, swallowing is more difficult, and the patient needs a period of retraining. Because the vocal folds remain intact and are functional, the patient can produce fairly normal voice.

b. **Indications for Use.** This procedure is used for tumors of the epiglottis and false vocal folds where the involvement is above the anterior commissure. Lesions should not extend into the base of tongue, pyriform sinus, or arytenoid body.

c. **Problems.** The technique produces good long-term survival while leaving intact vocal folds. Preservation of the true vocal folds is the primary distinction between this procedure and a

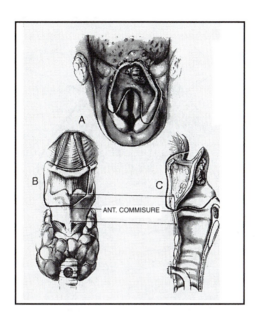

Figure 2–4. Areas removed after a supraglottic laryngectomy. A. Depicted is a lesion of the laryngeal side of the epiglottis. The area of resection is outlined in this supraglottic view, which includes the entire epiglottis, aryepiglottic fold, and false vocal cords. **B.** Anterior view outlining the line of resection, which includes the upper one half (upper one third in women and small men) of the thyroid cartilage on the side of the lesion and somewhat less on the contralateral side. **C.** Lateral view outlining the line of resection which passes through the base of the tongue above and through the ventricle below. (From Loré, J. M. [1988]. *An Atlas of Head and Neck Surgery* [3rd ed.]. Philadelphia: W. B. Saunders Company. Used by permission.)

total laryngectomy. Cure rates range from 75–90% or more. There have been some reports of delays in healing and fistula formation with the procedure. Swallowing problems are often present, requiring a period of retraining. Radiotherapy is equally effective for small supraglottic tumors. Because of a higher propensity of supraglottic tumors to metastasize to neck nodes, neck dissections are often done in conjunction with supraglottic laryngectomies.

3. Near Total Laryngectomy (Shunt)

a. Anatomic and Physiologic Changes. The entire larynx is removed with the exception of a narrow strip of tissue connecting the trachea with the pharynx above the uninvolved arytenoid (see Figure 2–5). This shunt is created from pieces of tissue from the larynx and, where necessary, from the pharynx.

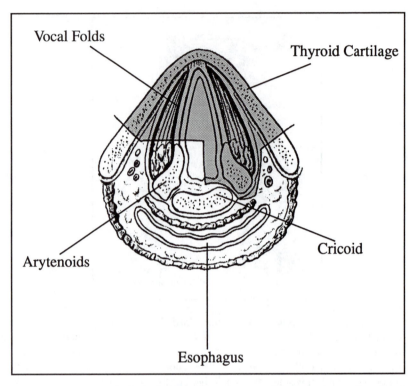

Figure 2–5. Areas removed (shaded area) after a near total laryngectomy. (Reprinted from Tucker, H. M. [1981]. *Surgery for Phonatory Disorders.* New York: Churchill Livingstone. Copyright 1981 by Cleveland Clinic Foundation. Used by permission.)

On the uninvolved side, the shunt is operated via intrinsic laryngeal muscle using the normal innervation. Voice is impaired as in a total laryngectomy, but because of the shunt, a form of voicing can be produced when the patient obstructs the tracheal opening and forces air up the tube formed by the shunt into the pharynx. Swallowing problems can be anticipated due to the removal of the structures that normally protect the airway.

b. **Indications for Use.** The procedure can be considered when the tumor does not involve the posterior commissure, one arytenoid, and one ventricle. It can be done in cases of extensive but unilateral transglottic, glottic, and advanced supraglottic cancers.

c. Pros and Cons. Potential problems include aspiration and stenosis (in about 20% of patients). Patients require training in swallowing and in sound production. In addition, some patients may experience problems in the shunt's functioning. Occasionally, completion of the laryngectomy needs to be done. The advantage of this technique is that it is possible to regain speech using the shunt, obviating the need for a prosthesis. Candidates must be carefully selected. The procedure does not eliminate the need for a total laryngectomy when the cancer extends beyond the acceptable borders. It cannot be used when both cords are fixed or when a posterior glottic lesion involving the interarytenoid region is present. Proper removal of all of the cancer should be the primary goal.

4. Total Laryngectomy

a. Anatomic and Physiologic Changes. The entire larynx is removed and removal may include the hyoid bone. The size and extent of resection into the pharynx is dependent on the extent of the tumor. The pharynx site is closed off, thus pulmonary air cannot be directed into the pharynx. Swallowing is generally not disturbed after internal healing is complete.

b. Indications for Use. Total laryngectomy is indicated when the initial cancer is extensive (T3 or T4) in cases of subglottic extension, or for salvage after radiation failure. Cure rates average 65–70% for T3 and 45–50% for T4 tumors.

c. Pros and Cons. Complications that may occur during and after the procedure include: carotid artery exposure, fistula formation, and edema. If the patient had preoperative irradiation, the surgery and postoperative healing may be more difficult. The advantage of the procedure is the higher cure rate for difficult carcinoma than radiotherapy alone. The patient experiences a loss of the ability to produce voice and needs to develop an alternative means of communication. The sense of smell may be altered. Swallowing and taste are generally preserved. With TE puncture, a means of phonation can be achieved.

5. Pharyngo-Laryngectomy

a. Anatomic and Physiologic Changes. This procedure is similar to a total laryngectomy except that parts of the pharynx must also be removed.

b. Indications for Use. The procedure needs to be considered when there is evidence of cancer in the pharyngeal region in addition to the larynx.

c. Pros and Cons. The problems are similar to those of total laryngectomy and perhaps slightly greater due to the more extensive surgical procedure. Loss of parts of the pharynx may limit options for the restoration of voice. Grafting of tissue may be required to replace excised tissue. Swallowing may pose a problem, particularly if there is stenosis at the esophageal inlet.

6. Composite Resection

a. Anatomic and Physiologic Changes. In a composite resection, several contiguous structures in the head or neck are removed. Thus, a laryngectomy with neck dissection would be considered a composite resection. The anatomic and physiological changes will vary depending on the structures removed.

b. Indications for Use. Extent of cancer and the degree of involvement of adjacent tissues will determine the need for this procedure. Evidence of cancer spread to the regional lymph nodes, musculature, or bone or cartilage or other structures in the neck would be positive indications for this procedure.

c. Pros and Cons. Extensive removal of adjacent tissue in the head and neck may pose problems for the patient. Swallowing, aspiration, and speech articulation, as well as phonation, may be affected. Where life itself may be threatened, the surgeon must remove all traces of the cancer and leave cancer-free margins. The goals of rehabilitation must be realistic and the patient fully informed about the limitations that will need to be faced after this procedure is performed.

7. Other Procedures

a. Esophageal Involvement. Occasionally, a tumor may extend into the esophagus, necessitating its partial removal. This procedure may interfere with swallowing and may limit the patient's alaryngeal speech options. The extent of esophageal resection will vary depending on the extent of the disease. Reconstruction can be obtained by a "gastric pullup" procedure or using a small intestine (jejunal) free-flap.

b. Tongue Involvement. Cancer of the larynx may also involve parts of the tongue, especially along the base of the tongue anterior to the hyoid. Parts of the tongue may need to be resected. The effect on speech will depend on the extent of the resection and the patient's subsequent ability to manipulate the tongue in production of speech. Because alaryngeal speech requires clarity of articulation, tongue resection can create serious problems in the acquisition of intelligible speech.

c. Radical Neck Dissection. Radical neck dissection refers to a surgical procedure in which the lymphatic system in the neck is removed to eliminate cancer cells that may have metastasized. It is performed if there is any clinical evidence of lymph metastases and it may be performed when there is a high likelihood of metastasis. The probability of metastasis increases as tumor size increases. In one study of 264 cases, it was found that metastasis occurred in about 2% of T1 glottic cases and rose to 65% in T4 glottic cases.

In addition to removal of the lymph nodes, the sternocleidomastoid muscle is often removed. This may interfere with neck rotation. Shoulder pain and a dropped shoulder may occur if the spinal accessory nerve has been sacrificed. Hypoglossal or facial nerve injury may result in speech/swallowing problems as well.

C. Combined Surgery and Radiation

1. When Used?

In some cases, a patient is given a course of irradiation after surgery to remove any small traces of the cancer. For many tumors, this course of irradiation increases survival (see Table 2–3). The major complications and sequelae of postoperative radiation are edema, difficulty swallowing, fatigue, thickened secretions, and soreness.

2. Indications for Use

Postoperative radiation may be indicated in surgery that attempts to salvage voice and swallowing and in an attempt to eradicate all vestiges of the cancer. In a total laryngectomy, radiation may be

Table 2–3. Five-year survival rates for surgery alone and surgery combined with irradiation.

Type/Stage of Cancer	Surgery Alone (%)	Surgery + Irradiation (%)
Supraglottic Stage IV	24	42
Glottic Stage III	53	50

Source: Adapted from Mendenhall, W. M., Parsons, J. T., Stringer, S. P., Cassisi, N. J., & Million, R. R. (1990). The role of radiation therapy in laryngeal cancer. *CA—A Cancer Journal for Clinicians, 40,* 150–156.

indicated for an advanced tumor, again to attempt to destroy cancer cells that may have begun to metastasize.

3. Timing of Procedure

Irradiation should commence after the patient has had a chance to heal but before there is a chance that tumor residue will begin growing.

D. Chemotherapy

1. Procedure

Chemotherapy may be used, like radiation, to reduce the chance of any residual tumor cells re-establishing themselves. Chemotherapy has been used only recently in tumors involving the larynx. It has been reported to assist in increasing the survival of patients with advanced disease.

2. Indications for Use

As was suggested for radiotherapy, chemotherapy may be indicated when the original tumor is large and there is a risk of metastasis.

3. Timing

Chemotherapy may be administered prior to or after surgery. A typical preoperative protocol might include 1 week of chemotherapy, followed by a 2-week rest, with another week of chemotherapy immediately prior to surgery. Postoperatively, chemotherapy may be given when the patient has healed sufficiently to tolerate the chemotherapy.

4. Problems

Some of the problems associated with chemotherapy are well known, including nausea, hair loss, weight loss, skin problems, and a deterioration of general body function.

E. Combined High-Dose Chemotherapy and Radiation

In patients with **advanced laryngeal cancer,** the combined use of high-dose chemotherapy and radiation therapy offers an alternative to surgical excision of the larynx. In one study, survival of combined radiotherapy and chemotherapy was equal to surgery and radiotherapy (68%), thereby preserving the patient's larynx. This approach has been driven by pretreatment consideration of potential functional loss of speech and swallowing. As stated by Weiss (1993, p. 312), "Quality of life counts for a great deal in the patients' minds. It should matter just as much to us."

IV. NEW DEVELOPMENTS

Refinements of existing surgical procedures are ongoing and research into improved procedures provides hope that conservation of the capacity to produce voicing without the assistance of any external or internal devices will be a reality at some future time. In 1969 a total laryngeal transplant in a human was performed in Belgium. That patient survived the surgery but died shortly thereafter. After a 19-year hiatus, a laryngeal transplant was performed in January 1998 by Dr. Marshall Strome of the Cleveland Clinic Foundation. The patient, a 40-year-old man whose larynx had been destroyed in a motorcycle accident 19 years previously, was reported to have spoken his first words 3 days postoperatively and continued to be able to speak in the following weeks.

There is much controversy in the medical community concerning the inherent risks of such a procedure and whether the benefits of producing voice and not having a stoma (if that turns out to be possible) outweigh the major life-threatening risks, such as a nonfunctional larynx with reinnervation (if it occurs at all) of incorrect muscle groups within the larynx, absence of the protective sphincteric mechanism of the supraglottic structures that prevent aspiration, questionable restoration of blood supply and the need for a repeat laryngectomy should that not occur, and the potential for organ rejection and infection due to the use of immunosuppressive drugs. Because the reporting of this event paralleled the revision date of this book, it is only possible to report the operation was done, the patient survived for at least 3 weeks and the patient could produce voice. Readers of this manual in future years will have to research the long-term outcome of this patient.

C H A P T E R

3

Total Rehabilitation of the Laryngectomee

I. GENERAL CONSIDERATIONS

Total rehabilitation of the laryngectomized individual requires the expertise of numerous specialists. The interaction of a multidisciplinary team should begin at the time that treatment for head and neck cancer is initiated. Rehabilitation planning begins at that time. "Few other cancers demonstrate the need for anticipatory treatment and rehabilitation to the magnitude required in the management of head and neck cancer" (Myers et al., 1986, p. 4). This chapter addresses the roles of those involved in the rehabilitation of the patient with special emphasis on the role of the speech-language pathologist. Although the role of the surgeon will not be addressed specifically, it must be understood that the surgeon is in charge of the team and carries the primary responsibility for the health care of the patient.

II. CONSIDERATIONS FOR THE SPEECH-LANGUAGE PATHOLOGIST

Many factors come into play during the initial contact between the speech-language pathologist and a person who is about to have, or may already have had, a total laryngectomy. These vary depending on when in the process from diagnosis to surgery the first contact takes place. However, some considerations are universal.

A. The "C" Word

The primary concern of all laryngectomees, and one that is never far below the surface no matter how many years pass, is the fear of cancer. Initially, there is the fear of not surviving the surgery. When that hurdle is passed, it is replaced by the dread that the surgeon may not have gotten "all of it" (the cancer). After the immediate concern blurs, a constant shadow remains—a fear of recurrence. Any lingering or new pain, unexpected bleeding, not feeling up to par, or anticipation of a routine visit to the doctor will sharpen that fear.

B. Loss of Control

As soon as an individual hears the diagnosis of cancer, there is a feeling that something has taken over his or her life—something over which the person has no control. The sense of loss of control is heightened as the need for various tests leads the person into new situations and strange environments where others control what happens. Suddenly, others tell you what you may or may not do, when you must do it, and where. There are few viable choices. It is important for the speech-language pathologist to recognize these feelings and to counteract them whenever possible by encouraging the individual to exercise control through making choices regarding communication. The person must be made aware of the responsibilities he or she must assume relative to communication.

C. Prognostic Factors

The overall prognosis for survival of laryngeal cancer, as discussed in Chapter 1 (Table 1–2), is relatively good. However, this depends on the type, location, invasiveness, and spread of the disease. Clearly, the sooner the cancer is detected, the better the prognosis for survival. The prognosis for recovery of speech function also depends on a number of factors that co-exist and interact in a complex manner. Although the following sections will address many of those factors individually, the clinician should not lose sight of the probability that there is more than a single factor involved in determination of prognosis.

1. Data about the **effect of age on rehabilitation outcome** are minimal. We know that biological aging is more significant than chronological aging. Thus, we are concerned with age as it relates to the individual's overall status and functional level. An individual's need and desire to communicate, however, cannot be determined by age alone. The speech-language pathologist must guard against making prognostic judgments based solely on age.

2. The **extent of surgery** the patient has had must be considered. The more extensive the disease at the time of diagnosis, the more likelihood there is of spread or metastasis; clearly, a negative factor for long-term survival. The prognosis for acquisition of speech may also be influenced negatively by extensive disease. Large invasive tumors may necessitate extensive surgery and a lengthier and more complicated hospital course. If major reconstruction of pharyngeal and/or esophageal defects is required, the acquisition of esophageal speech may be compromised. It is not the case, however, that it can never be learned. We have worked with persons who have had extensive reconstruction procedures along with total laryngectomy yet have, with great determination, mastered esophageal speech. Surgical prosthetic voice restoration can still be an option even when the extent of surgery has been great, but voice quality and clarity of speech may be poorer than might otherwise be the case. When surgical resection of significant portions of the tongue has been necessary, the acquisition of any form of intelligible alaryngeal speech will be problematic because of the constraints imposed on the person's ability to articulate. However, prosthetic alteration of oral contour (such as an augmentative palatal prostheses) and other means of communication (augmentative communication systems) will still be available and should be pursued.

3. Previous research has shown a high negative correlation between **hearing impairment** and acquisition of alaryngeal speech (Diedrich & Youngstrom, 1966). The presence of significant hearing loss, particularly when not compensated by the use of amplification, has a negative influence on the person's ability to acquire good esophageal speech and, indeed, negatively affects the quality and clarity of any mode of alaryngeal speech. Our clinical experience confirms this. Patients who have significant hearing losses and

refuse to wear amplification cannot appreciate the model of speech presented to them, cannot monitor their own productions adequately, and often produce excessive stoma blast accompanying speech attempts of all types. Clarity of articulation also suffers, because the patient is unable to hear the production of voiceless consonants and does not produce them accurately.

4. Attempts have been made to correlate **personality type** or characteristics with response to rehabilitation. However, human beings are not simple or predictable. The temptation to predict outcome based on characterization of a patient's personality type, for example, dependent, weak, anxious, hostile, and so forth, should be tempered. All of us who work with people would agree that personality factors cannot be ignored, but what we cannot predict is the specific effect of having a laryngectomy on a given individual, the influences that may motivate the person toward a goal, or the forces that may make laryngectomy an insurmountable trauma. We have seen people overcome their postoperative voiceless state and their initial depression to become vocal advocates for others and take on leadership roles they had never previously imagined even with an intact larynx. And, we have also known those who proclaim all to be well, give lip service to their determination, only to succumb to deep despair and depression. In the presence of despair, depression, and extreme anxiety, the prognosis for successful rehabilitation, including successful acquisition of a new mode of speech, suffers greatly. It is incumbent on the speech-language pathologist to recognize these conditions, be aware of their potential effect on the patient's progress, and refer the patient for appropriate counseling.

5. Medical/surgical treatment protocols often require the patient to have an extensive course of **radiation therapy** following surgery. This may require daily treatments for 5 to 6 weeks. These treatments often run concurrently with speech therapy and may have a negative impact on the patient's progress in acquiring a new speech mode, particularly esophageal speech. Thus, a lengthier course of speech therapy may be anticipated. However, time is not the only by-product of radiation therapy that must be considered. Patients respond to radiation in an individual manner. Some of the physical effects may be: fatigue, sore throat, dry mouth, thickened mucus, and dental and gum changes that may result in ill-fitting dentures. All of these may interfere, at least temporarily, with the acquisition of alaryngeal speech. In addition, there are psychological effects that cannot be ignored and may have a pro-

foundly negative impact on prognosis for rehabilitation. The patient has recently had major surgery, physical stamina may still be compromised as a result, adjustment to and acceptance of the changes brought about by the surgery are in the earliest stage, and the ability to speak has not yet been established. To these considerations, add the physical effects noted before. The totality of these concerns can have a potentially devastating effect. Many patients may cease attending speech therapy during this time and, indeed, may be lost to follow-up. Those who can and do continue to receive speech therapy may make limited progress and can become depressed. They need support from the speech-language pathologist, from other laryngectomees, and from their families. Although the effects of radiation therapy on prognosis for speech are generally negative in the short term, there is no evidence that there are lasting effects that have a seriously negative impact on long-term prognosis for speech learning.

6. Although a patient's **cognitive status** must be taken into account, premature negative judgments about the ability to learn a new mode of speech must be avoided. We have worked with patients who carried the diagnosis of developmental delay, yet they acquired very acceptable alaryngeal speech, including esophageal speech. Others have had difficulty managing any mode of alaryngeal speech. The speech-language pathologist must have sufficient skill and flexibility to adapt the teaching approach to the patient's needs and learning style. Patients with cognitive deficits resulting from stroke, traumatic brain injury, or other degenerative neurological diseases who require laryngeal amputation present a difficult challenge. Their prognosis for acquiring any mode of alaryngeal speech is guarded and will depend on the results of a thorough assessment of their linguistic and oromotor abilities. With this group of patients, the speech-language pathologist must find the most effective means of communication, verbal or nonverbal. If the speech-language pathologist skilled in alaryngeal communication determines that the patient is incapable of acquiring mechanical, esophageal, or prosthetically aided speech, referral should be made for assessment with other augmentative/alternative communication systems.

7. The **skill of the speech-language pathologist influences prognosis**. We believe strict adherence to the Code of Ethics of the American-Speech-Language-Hearing Association is necessary. The Code states that "Individuals shall engage in only those aspects of the professions that are within the scope of their com-

petence considering their level of education, training, and experience." And further, "Individuals shall prohibit any of their professional staff from providing services that exceed the staff member's competence considering the staff member's level of education, training, and experience" (American Speech-Language-Hearing Association, 1994, Code of ethics. *Asha, 36*[Suppl. 13], pp. 1–2). The teaching of alaryngeal speech requires specialized training, knowledge, and skill. In the absence of such qualifications, the outcome for the patient may be compromised.

III. ROLE OF THE SPEECH-LANGUAGE PATHOLOGIST

A. Preoperative Consultation

A preoperative consultation is essential. Referral for preoperative consultation is made by the surgeon and, ideally, should take place soon after the physician has made the diagnosis and has met with the patient to discuss the findings and the recommendation for surgery. Although the timing of this consultation depends on when referral is made, whenever possible, it should take place in the speech pathologist's office prior to hospital admission. As soon as the patient enters the hospital, subtle changes occur that involve the loss of control discussed previously. Furthermore, due to the highly controlled limitations on hospital stays, patients are usually admitted to the hospital on the eve or day of the scheduled surgery and immediately overloaded with information from physicians, nurses, dietitians, anesthesiologists, and others. This makes it an inauspicious time to talk to patients about communication. However, there are times when the option for preoperative consultation outside of the hospital does not exist. It is still essential for the speech-language pathologist to meet with the patient, and, perhaps, temper the amount of information that is provided. The patient will have a limited time to absorb new information. It is beneficial for immediate family members, close friends, or caregivers (persons of the patient's choosing) to be present during this consultation. The more they understand about the surgery, what to expect in the immediate postoperative period, the anticipated hospital course, and the rehabilitation options, the more support they will be able to provide to the patient.

1. There are a number of ways in which the preoperative consultation is of **value to the patient** and to those who will be providing ongoing support.

a. They are **ready to "hear" more** now that they have had some time to deal with the knowledge that cancer is present. Patients often recall relatively little of what they are initially told by their doctors when that information is paired with learning the diagnosis. Time spent in talking with the speech-language pathologist offers the opportunity to:

   (1) review what the patient knows,
   (2) correct any misunderstandings,
   (3) reinforce essential information,
   (4) provide new information,
   (5) allow time for questions, and
   (6) discuss communication options.

b. The speech-language pathologist must exercise sensitivity in **assessing how much information the patient is prepared to hear**. This does not mean the speech-language pathologist should withhold information if the patient wants it. We tell our patients what we can offer and allow them to tell us how much they are interested in hearing.

   (1) Talk about the **speech options** that may be available to them.
   (2) Offer the **opportunity to see, hear, or have demonstrated** any, or all, of the speech types and proceed only as far as patients wish to go. If they choose not to hear the various types of speech preoperatively, they will have that opportunity after their surgery.
   (3) If time permits, offer the **option to meet a laryngectomized individual** who has mastered alaryngeal speech.
   (4) It is also important for the speech-language pathologist to be cognizant of, and sensitive to, the **practices of referring physicians**. Some may be strong advocates of a trial of esophageal speech training prior to consideration of surgical prosthetic voice restoration. Others prefer to proceed with tracheoesophageal puncture at the time of the laryngectomy. Patients must have faith in their surgeons, and that must never be undermined, or seem to be undermined, by presenting choices to a patient that, in fact, may not be consistent with the surgeon's advice.
   (5) The speech-language pathologist should **discuss all information or concerns** that may influence a patient's treatment **with the surgeon**.
   (6) In this preoperative consultation with the speech-language pathologist, the patient has the **opportunity to make direct**

contact with the person who will be helping him or her after the surgery. This is reassuring at this stage, and it eases the postoperative contacts when a known face appears at the bedside.

2. The preoperative consultation also has **value for the speech-language pathologist**.

   a. It is **easier to communicate** with an individual who still has a larynx and has not just had major surgery than with one who is trying to deal with pain, discomfort, voicelessness, and perhaps an annoying tube in the nose. Thus, the nature of the relationship that is established preoperatively will be different from the one that begins after surgery.

   b. It is also valuable to **hear the person's habitual speech style**. We recall our initial consultation with a gentleman who had a pronounced Scottish brogue which made it difficult for us to understand him. If we had not heard his speech pattern preoperatively, we would have had a difficult time trying to figure out what was going on with his alaryngeal speech. In another instance, a patient had severe hypernasality and extremely distorted sound productions due to a poorly repaired cleft palate. In less extreme cases, it is also valuable to hear the patient's speech pattern. We learn whether this is someone who speaks clearly or who tends to mumble, or someone who speaks rapidly with nonstop sentences, or a person of few words. These observations have implications for areas that may need special attention in the teaching of alaryngeal speech.

   c. The speech-language pathologist can **obtain a representative sample of the patient's cognitive status** through discussion and screening testing.

   d. The speech-language pathologist **should obtain a sample of the patient's writing** to assess whether that will be a viable mode of communication during the immediate postoperative period.

   e. If possible, **audiological assessment** can be carried out during the preoperative visit. Otherwise, such testing should be done when the patient begins alaryngeal speech training.

B. Postoperative Consultation

The nature of this contact will depend on whether the patient had been seen prior to surgery, whether this contact takes place in the hospital or following discharge, and whether surgical prosthetic voice restoration has already begun or is planned. It is highly recommended that family members or close friends be present during this consultation. They can be more supportive and helpful to the laryngectomee when they are informed. It is important that they be included from the start, so that they can assist the patient in developing alaryngeal speech. The speech-language pathologist must be sensitive to negative reactions by family members or friends which, if not addressed, may sabotage the patient's early speech attempts.

1. If this is the **first contact with the patient** and it takes place in the hospital, the speech-language pathologist should ascertain what the patient knows about his or her condition and what the expectations are concerning speech. It is not necessary to cover all the material that might have been included in a presurgical contact, because the patient has already gone through the surgery and is now ready to go beyond it. If a tracheoesophageal puncture has been performed or is planned in the immediate future, the discussion about communication should focus on that. However, in these instances, temporary use of an oral type of electronic speech aid may be helpful and should, therefore, be a part of the discussion. The patient should be given the opportunity to talk with a laryngectomized person who is successfully using tracheoesophageal speech.

2. If the patient was seen preoperatively, the **follow-up contact** should take place after the patient is out of intensive care and has returned to the floor where recovery will continue. As the length of hospitalization following surgery has shortened, it has become necessary for patients to be seen earlier in their recovery course than might, on occasion, be ideal. The speech-language pathologist should make the determination relative to the patient's readiness to deal with a speech aid and should not impose this on a patient who is incapable of dealing with it either physically or emotionally. It may, in some instances, be more productive to postpone introduction of the device for a few days. The speech-language pathologist must be cognizant of the practices and preferences of the specific hospital and its physicians concerning the need for medical clearance for follow-up visits. In many settings,

it is expected that once you have become involved with a case, you will follow that case without the need for further medical clearance. However, if there is any uncertainty about the nature of the surgery that was performed, the status of the healing process, or about the patient's general condition, the speech-language pathologist should contact the surgeon prior to instituting any course of rehabilitation. In all cases, the speech-language pathologist should review the medical chart prior to visiting the patient to determine whether postoperative problems have been encountered that might negate a visit at that time or require postponement of initiation of alaryngeal speech.

3. The **content of the follow-up visit** should include:

   a. **Review of the earlier discussion**, including the modes of alaryngeal speech (unless, as noted above, the patient will be using tracheoesophageal speech).

   b. If not previously done, a **demonstration of electronic speech aids** can be given. Although most patients are not ready to use a neck-held type of instrument so soon after surgery, they should be made aware of them as a possible future option.

   c. Depending on the patient's condition and readiness, **teach the use of an oral type of instrument at this time**. A loaner instrument can be provided for the patient's use in the hospital. Another option would be to dispense a speech aid to the patient. In that instance, it is advisable to dispense an instrument that can be purchased with an oral adapter. Thus, the patient will have the option of using it as a neck-held instrument, if appropriate, after swelling has resolved. If loaner instruments are not available or the choice of alaryngeal speech mode is uncertain, the inexpensive and disposable P.O.Vox unit (see Chapter 4 and Appendix D) can be dispensed to the patient.

   d. Arrange a **visit by a previously laryngectomized individual** unless the patient objects or has previously had such contact.

   e. It is appropriate at this time to **discuss rehabilitation plans**. The specific content of this discussion will, once again, be determined by choices that have been made regarding the alaryngeal speech mode. Generally, patients should be advised when they will be seen again, where they will be seen, by whom, and for what. Names, addresses, phone numbers, and appointment times should be provided in writing. The first question universally raised by patients, and often the most difficult to answer, concerns the length of time it will take for them to learn a new mode of speech. It is essential that the speech-language pathologist be encouraging without making promises that may not be deliverable. Statements such as, "We'll have you talking in no time!" should be avoided.

f. It is helpful to leave **written information** that the patient and others may review and refer to along the way. The American Cancer Society provides kits of informative material free of charge. These can be extremely helpful, but they must be checked periodically to ensure they are current and accurate. (See Appendix E.) Various methods of dissemination may be used: they may be given to the patient by the speech-language pathologist during either the pre- or postoperative consultation, they may be disseminated by a laryngectomee visitor, or they may be provided by the nursing staff at the time of the patient's admission to the hospital. Our preference is to provide kits when we talk with the patient about the information. At the very least, we hope the kits are distributed by a knowledgeable person who can provide guidance about the materials.

C. Use of the Rehabilitated Laryngectomee and Support Groups

1. The rehabilitated laryngectomee can provide a valuable type of support. Persons who share a common experience or concern are able to provide support to each other that is different from what is offered by those who do not share that common bond. Thus, the opportunity to meet and talk with a previously laryngectomized person who has learned a mode of alaryngeal speech and has made a good adjustment can be invaluable to the person who is entering this group.

a. The **timing of such a visit** may be determined by: the stage at which initial referral occurs; the patient's previous exposure to, or friendship with, laryngectomized individuals; the patient's readiness to pursue such a visit; and the availability of appropriate volunteers to provide such visits. Some surgeons have one or two patients they ask to visit new patients. When that is not the case, the speech-language pathologist often assumes the responsibility for making the connection. In some areas, there may be an active support group that provides visitation as a service, and the local Cancer Society may be the resource in other areas. The speech-language pathologist should be aware of the resources available and make use of them.

b. Although there is no controversy about the value of such visits, there may be some as to what constitutes an **appropriate visitor**. Ideally, the visitor should be well trained in the "art" of visitation and should be matched to the person to be visited in gender, age, employment status, and type of alaryngeal speech used. Although this is not always possible, these are goals that can be pursued. The art of visiting includes the ability to subordinate concern about oneself and one's own experience to the ability to listen to another; to understand those areas that should not be discussed by lay persons; and to play a supportive role. We know an accomplished esophageal speaker who told newly laryngectomized persons that it only took him 4 days to learn to talk (esophageal speech) and that he did it by himself. This not only raises inappropriate expectations, but also may lead to depression and a sense of failure if those expectations are not met.

2. Organized **support groups** serve a variety of purposes, but they vary in their programs. Some offer speech training, others offer an opportunity to practice speech being newly acquired; some offer informational types of programs, others may be primarily social in nature; some offer separate support for families, others offer a place for all to talk together; some become involved in visitor training and sponsoring a visitation program, others may provide a list of members who are available to be called on but without specific training; some become involved in community education as speakers about cancer; and, in some instances, laryngectomees will be involved in cancer support groups that are not restricted to those with laryngeal cancer. (See Appendix C for names of organizations and associations.) It should also be mentioned that the Internet has become a valuable source of information and support. There are numerous sites, including an online chat group. Addresses for these can be found in Appendix G.

D. Psychosocial Considerations

We have already discussed some of the psychosocial implications for the person who has been diagnosed with laryngeal cancer and faces the prospect of removal of the larynx with the concomitant loss of the ability to speak. In addition to the fear of cancer and the immediate concern about survival, other concerns begin to arise, for example, economic concerns, loss of identity, issues of self-image, reactions of family and friends, reactions of others, and sexual concerns. Many of these may not seem to have direct significance for the speech-language pathologist; however, unresolved issues can hinder a patient's ability to benefit from rehabilitation efforts. It is the responsibility of the speech-language pathologist to be aware of these problems; to provide a supportive, open, nonjudgmental atmosphere in which they can be discussed; and to offer referral to appropriate personnel or agencies. (See Section E in this chapter for discussion of the role of the social worker on the rehabilitation team.)

1. **Economic concerns** often arise early for the individual diagnosed with laryngeal cancer. These are usually twofold. First, there is the immediate concern about the cost of medical/surgical care. This is followed by uncertainty about future earning power, or for the retired person, concern about the adequacy of retirement income to meet increased medical needs. These concerns may be apparent very early and evidenced by the individual's questions about the cost of speech therapy and electronic speech aids during the pre- or postoperative consultations. However, a patient's lack of verbalized concern should not be construed to mean that there is an absence of concern. It is an area that may need to be explored in a very sensitive manner so that all available sources of assistance can be offered. The speech-language pathologist should be knowledgeable about some of the sources of third party support that patients may access (e.g., Medicare, Medicaid, private insurance); about support from local service clubs (e.g., Rotary, Lions, Sertoma); or about support from the local cancer society that may provide assistance with transportation or medical equipment. The rehabilitation team social worker is an invaluable resource for these types of concerns.

2. The loss of voice and ability to communicate is closely bound to a sense of **loss of identity**. We use communication to shape our environment; establish our status and position; and state our ideas, thoughts, and approval or lack thereof. Even the sound of our voice is part of our identity. There is understandable mourning and grieving for the loss of that identity. Even though a means of communication may be regained, the person will be changed. Some who were dominant in their role in the family, at work, and with friends may now feel helpless and dependent. Such feelings

lead to frustration and easy irritation. In turn, family members, friends, and co-workers may resent the changed roles and expectations and reveal their own frustration and irritation. Recognition of these dynamics by those involved with the individual, that is, families, friends, and professionals, as well as by the patient, is vital. The speech-language pathologist must help the patient and the family acknowledge and understand these feelings by providing an open, accepting atmosphere in which honest discussion can take place. Patients need the opportunity to express these concerns where they will be heard without judgment, without being brushed aside, and perhaps with the input from others who have had similar experience. The speech-language pathologist must also be sensitive to the need for referring the patient for appropriate counseling.

3. Obvious changes in physical appearance have a deep effect on **self-image**. The presence of the stoma, obvious scarring, and differences in the contour of the neck are readily observable changes. Add to those the changes in respiratory sounds and the sound of the cough, the need to cover and clean the stoma after coughing, and the effects of a laryngectomy on self-image become readily apparent. Beyond that, we must recognize how much our feelings about our image affect our functioning. Once again, these are feelings that must be aired and discussed with others who have experienced them. In the absence of a group setting, the speech-language pathologist must use extreme skill in making it possible for the patient to talk about these issues in an honest and open way. Referral should be an option if the patient appears to be having difficulty in making an adjustment. If the patient has not previously been counseled about the need to keep the stoma covered at all times, this may fall to the speech-language pathologist. The patient's self-image may be enhanced by the use of various types of stoma coverings, not only the most traditional crocheted variety.

4. The **reactions of family and friends** to the diagnosis of cancer, and subsequently to the postsurgical changes in appearance and function, must be considered and understood. Too often, people react as if the diagnosis of cancer is a terminal diagnosis. Such a belief makes many uncomfortable in the presence of the person who has been given the diagnosis. It is important that a more realistic understanding of the diagnosis be explained to the family. Usually, this is done by the physician at the time that the diagnosis is made. However, because patients and family members may

not fully recall or comprehend the physician's explanation, it may need to be repeated several times. Because of the physiological changes, as well as the lost or changed ability to communicate, laryngectomized persons often fear and dread re-entry into their social circles. For some individuals, any evidence of discomfort on the part of friends, any difficulty in communication, can be enough to result in withdrawal from such contacts. Such reactions can result in depression and erosion of feelings of self-worth. As a patient's ability to communicate progresses, the speech-language pathologist should incorporate therapeutic activities that require interaction with persons outside of the therapy setting while providing the support that can make it possible for the patient to experience success. Helping the patient and family to manipulate their environment to permit gradual "re-entry" can be most beneficial. For example, one or two people with whom they feel most at ease can be invited for a brief visit. Patients need to be encouraged to express their fears and anxieties openly to these friends and to educate them in how they can be helpful. We encourage patients to let family members and friends know that their attempts at speaking are not painful, that they cannot speak quickly, and that they appreciate being told honestly when they are not understood.

5. Persons who make a good initial adjustment with family and close friends may fear the **reactions of others**, thus finding it difficult to extend beyond that closed circle. A type of helplessness and dependency on others may emerge that can be frustrating to all. Such feelings also feed erosion of self-worth and depression. Recognition of such reactions is the first step in dealing with them and getting beyond them.

6. The **frustrations of learning to talk** again are complicated and real. Those who have successful surgical-prosthetic voice restoration have the shortest period of such frustration. For others, it may be protracted. We have observed that there is often a reversion to, or a reliving of, school experiences. Because learning to talk is something we associate with childhood, the need to do this as an adult has complex ramifications. People react much as they might have when they were school children. They make excuses for not practicing, or they lie about whether they have "done their homework." They freeze in therapy when they are trying to "show off to the teacher," protesting how well they can do at home. The speech-language pathologist must be aware of these feelings and attempt to counteract them by always treating patients as the

adults they are. We address all adult patients by the appropriate title (Mr., Ms., etc.) and last name. This seems to promote feelings of identity and self-worth.

7. Too often, the area of **sexual concerns** is ignored or avoided by most professionals involved in the rehabilitation of the laryngectomee. Rarely will the laryngectomee raise the topic even though he or she is concerned. Some of that concern results from the change in self-image and concern about the partner's reaction to the physical changes. Some has to do with the changed breathing patterns and worry about needing to cough or having mucus expelled from the stoma. There are ways to deal with all of these concerns. The first is to talk about them. Patients may need the help of a professional in being able to do so. One patient told us that there really was not a problem as long as the partners were willing to change positions. Another recalled that after her surgery her husband seemed to be very distant until she told him that the doctor had only removed her larynx and had not altered any other part of her anatomy.

E. Role of the Social Worker

A social worker can be an invaluable asset to the rehabilitation team that serves the needs of laryngectomized patients and their families. If such a team does not exist, the speech-language pathologist should make every effort to establish a close working relationship with an interested social worker. Most hospitals have social workers or care coordinators (RNs) on staff to assist patients with financial arrangements and with discharge planning, including the need for any specialized pieces of home equipment such as suction machines, with transportation arrangements for medical appointments, and so forth.

1. **The social worker's value** to the team is great. It is helpful to have the social worker meet with the patient and any accompanying person during the patient's first visit. Time can be devoted to issues that might otherwise be ignored, information can be elicited, and assistance can be provided in ways that are beyond the speech-language pathologist's competence. The social worker maintains contact with both the patient and the family throughout the course of therapy and sometimes beyond meeting with family members while the patient is receiving speech therapy. Because support of family members and friends in the rehabilitation process is so important, the social worker's ability to elicit that support is invaluable. Our experience is that the psychosocial

concerns discussed in the previous section are expertly addressed by the social worker in ongoing contacts with the patients.

F. Other Members of the Rehabilitation Team

The case can be made for including many other health care workers in the rehabilitation team.

1. Clearly, **nurses** play a major role during hospitalization. They are not only involved in the day-to-day care of the patient, but also teach new self-care practices, for example, how to clean the stoma, how to change dressings if needed, and how to use the suction machine. They must address general hygiene needs, particularly in the probable presence of a reduction in the patient's sense of smell. They see the patient through the most difficult postsurgical period. Nurses need to be aware of the role of the speech-language pathologist and of the various alaryngeal speech modalities. If a patient begins to use an electronic speech aid during the hospital stay, the nurse can be very helpful in taking the time to listen and be supportive. Knowledge about the instruments and familiarity with how they work enhances the nurse's ability to provide this assistance. The speech-language pathologist should provide instruction to nursing staff through inservice presentations and individual contacts.

2. Patients who have had radical neck dissection with sacrifice of the spinal accessory nerve may benefit from the services of a **physical therapist**. The dropping of the shoulder on the affected side may result in limited range of movement if appropriate exercise is not provided. Also, patients may complain of pain, which can be reduced with physical therapy.

3. Nutritionists, psychologists, and vocational counselors may be helpful in various aspects of the rehabilitation process. Although our team does not include all of these professionals, they are available on referral and should be utilized to provide specific assistance when it would be helpful to the patient.

4. Patients frequently require the attention of a **dentist and/or prosthodontist** following surgery and particularly following radiation therapy. Teeth that are in the field receiving irradiation are often lost. Because tissues may shrink following radiation, patients may find that their dentures no longer fit and require either replacement or adjustment. The absence of teeth may have a detrimental effect on the clarity of articulation of alaryngeal speech.

G. Special Considerations for Hospitalization or Emergency Care of Laryngectomees

Because the speech-language pathologist is often the professional who provides information to the patient, family, and caregivers relative to many of the needs and concerns of a laryngectomee, we believe that inclusion of information about special considerations in the event of emergency or future hospitalizations is appropriate here.

At the time of laryngectomy the individual is cared for by nurses skilled in the care of head and neck surgical patients. However, it may be necessary for the now laryngectomized person to be hospitalized for other illness or surgeries that would place him or her in a different area of the hospital or a different hospital where the personnel are not as knowledgable about the needs of the laryngectomee. Because there are respiratory and communication needs that are unique to the laryngectomee, it is beneficial for the patient and others to be aware of these needs and how they should be handled. A guideline for this can be found in Appendix A.

A videotape, "Check the Neck" (available from the International Association of Laryngectomees [IAL]), provides excellent information on rescue breathing for the laryngectomized person or any other person who depends on ventilation via tracheostoma. It is approved by the American Cancer Society and the American Red Cross. Contact your local ACS association for availability of this tape. During a crisis, giving oxygen to a laryngectomized person improperly via a face mask rather than correctly at the stoma can result in brain damage or death.

It is clear that total rehabilitation of the person who has had surgical removal of the larynx is a complex process that involves professionals from numerous disciplines, the patient, his or her family and/or friends, and supportive people who have been through the experience. It has been stated that "the goal of integrating treatment and rehabilitation is to prevent or minimize the physical (cosmetic or functional) disability and the emotional sequelae commonly associated with head and neck cancer and its treatment" (Myers et al., 1986, p. 4). One major goal of the process is to have the individual return to his or her former life-style and routine with a means of communication that satisfactorily fulfills social, emotional, and vocational needs. "When internal or external body parts that contribute to functions or features are lost from the whole, a person is immeasurably diminished. Successful rehabilitation, then, must have its focus not on what has been lost, but on how to restore function and appearance to what remains" (Blitzer et al., 1985, p. ix).

CHAPTER

4

Alaryngeal Speech

After removal of the larynx, the patient no longer has a source of sound for speaking. Fortunately, there are a variety of devices and procedures that can provide a new source of sound. The patient can then use his or her articulators to produce the sounds of speech. There are two general categories of sound source restoration—mechanical speech aids and alternative "natural" sound sources. In the former category are the pneumatic and electronic external sound sources and in the latter are esophageal and tracheoesophageal speech. Advantages and disadvantages of each form of alaryngeal speech are presented in Table 4–1. The various mechanical speech aids and voice prostheses are discussed in the following sections. A list of manufacturers and suppliers of alaryngeal devices is provided in Appendix D.

I. PNEUMATIC DEVICES

A. Description

Pneumatic speech devices were among the first to be used as replacements for voice production and are still in use today. They usually consist of a piece that fits over the stoma, a small unit with

Table 4–1. Comparison of alaryngeal speech modes.

Type of Speech	Advantages	Disadvantages
Pneumatic speech aid	"natural" nonelectronic sound easy to learn intelligible speech inexpensive initial cost inexpensive operating cost (no batteries)	bulky size requires access to stoma sometimes difficult to maintain seal at stoma

Electronic speech aid
(Neck type)
	easy to learn to use
	fits in pocket or purse
	volume and pitch controls
	    for individual preference
	adequate volume to be
	    heard in noisy places
	intelligible speech when
	    used well
		noisy electronic sound
		cannot be used with heavily
		    scarred or erythematous
		    neck
		moderate initial cost
		occasional extra cost for
		    repair
		requires very clear articulation
		    skills

Electronic speech aid
(Oral type)
	easy to learn to use
	fits in pocket or purse, but
	    may be larger than neck
	    type
	volume and pitch controls
	    for individual preference
	adequate volume to be heard
	    in noisy places
	may be less noisy than neck
	    types (with or without oral
	    adapter)
	can be used soon after
	    surgery even in presence
	    of much scar tissue
	intelligible when used well
		electronic sound
		    very obvious to all
		    observers
		"clumsy" feeling initially to
		    talk with tube in mouth
		moderate initial purchase
		    cost
		occasional additional cost
		    for repairs
		requires excellent
		    articulation skill for easy
		    intelligibility

Esophageal speech	"natural" nonelectronic
	    sound
	requires no dependence on
	    mechanical instrument
	    or other device
	sound of the voice does not
	    call attention to itself
	    (may be perceived as
	    having a cold)
		a period of therapy required
		    for most people
		may be difficult for one
		    third or more patients to
		    learn well enough to be
		    easily intelligible
		difficult to hear in noisy
		    environments
		requires excellent
		    articulation skills
		may exacerbate symptoms
		    of gastroesophageal reflux
		    continued

Table 4–1. (*continued*)

Type of Speech	Advantages	Disadvantages
Tracheoesophageal speech	"natural" nonelectronic sound requires short learning period smooth, fluent speech using long sentences because of availability of pulmonary air flexibility of loudness and pitch variations sound of the voice does not call attention to itself extended wear prosthesis types obviate need for frequent removal	if not done as primary procedure, requires another surgical procedure requires manual dexterity, visual acuity, and level of alertness to care for requires use of finger to occlude stoma or daily affixing of valve to peristomal area buildup of candida deposits requiring frequent cleaning

a reed inside to provide the sound, and tubing that carries the sound to the mouth. The patient places the tube in the corner of his or her mouth as exhalatory air from the lungs drives the reed to produce sound that is resonated in the usual way in the patient's oral cavity and shaped into words by the action of the articulators.

B. Specific Types

1. DSP8 Speech Aid

In this device, the vibrator is housed within the tubing. It is relatively inexpensive and is available from Memacon in the Netherlands.

2. Tokyo Speech Aid

This device (Figure 4–1) is another relatively inexpensive unit and is supplied with a training tape. The tone generating mechanism is made of a thin, soft material that is self-cut and placed in the housing. It is replaced as necessary.

3. ToneAire Artificial Larynx

This is a new product that is also relatively inexpensive. The ToneAire has a metal reed mechanism in the sound chamber

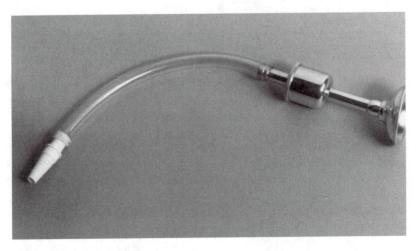

Figure 4–1. The Tokyo speech aid.

that is not removed. The angle of the air tube can be customized by bending it to the specific mouth-to-stoma characteristics of the individual so that it fits directly into the speaker's mouth as the sound chamber is held to the stoma. This allows the unit to be held with only one hand.

C. Advantages

The two major advantages of pneumatic devices are that they do not have a buzzing electronic sound and that they use the patient's own pulmonary air supply. Phonation can be easily coordinated with respiration and loud voice can be produced. The patient can use his or her normal phrasing and flow of speech without the need to turn an oscillator on and off.

D. Disadvantages

There are several problems with the pneumatic devices. First, they require access to the stoma for placement of the instrument. Most patients typically wear some kind of covering over the stoma, making access to it awkward. Second, the devices require the use of at least one hand, thus limiting the patient's ability to perform tasks requiring the use of both hands. Third, they are visually distracting to the listener. Other problems include the lack of pitch control and the low fundamental frequency, which may be a problem for a female user.

II. ELECTRONIC DEVICES

A. Description

These devices use electric power to drive a vibrator that provides the sound source. One version of these devices consists of a tube attached to the electrically powered vibrator. The tube fits inside the mouth in much the same way as in the pneumatic devices. Sound delivered into the oral cavity is articulated in the normal way. Another version consists of a hand held vibrator that is designed to deliver the sound through the skin when placed on the neck. A third type is contained in a dental plate worn by the patient and activated by a hand held unit.

There are numerous manufacturers who produce electronic speech aids powered by batteries. The differences among the various models of these aids are appearance, size, quality of sound, ability to change pitch and loudness characteristics, and the types of batteries required.

B. Specific Types

The following is a representative sampling of some of the instruments currently in use. This is not meant to be an exhaustive list and is purely descriptive in nature. The order in which the instruments are listed should not be construed to denote a ranking or preference. The choice of an instrument must be governed by what is best for each individual and is best done with the guidance of a skilled speech-language pathologist.

1. Cooper-Rand Electronic Speech Aid

This device, manufactured by Luminaud, is a battery-powered sound source that directs the sound into the oral cavity via a small tube placed in the mouth. It is the only instrument that is designed to be used exclusively as an oral device (Figure 4–2). Oral placement may be advantageous immediately after surgery, because the patient can use it without interfering with neck healing or causing discomfort. The unit is lightweight (about 7 oz) and can be carried in a shirt or blouse pocket. An extra long cord (40 in) permits placing the device in other locations as well, such as on a table or a bed. The unit is controlled from the push button on the tone generator to which the oral

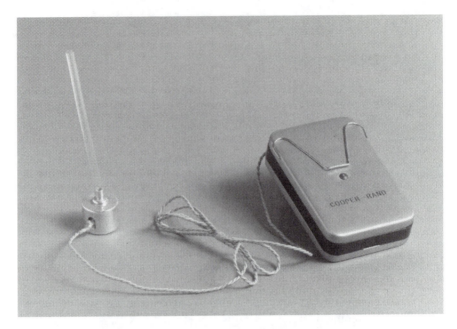

Figure 4–2. The Cooper-Rand electronic speech aid.

tube is attached. The company offers several options that address a variety of patients' needs, for example, varying lengths of connecting cords, an extended grip tone generator model (see Figure 4–3) that allows for easier handling, and a "no-hands" model that uses alternative modes of tone generation. The unit is powered by two 9-volt alkaline batteries which last 4–6 weeks. Pitch and volume controls provide limited variation of these parameters. The cord that connects the tone generator to the unit requires replacement very few months. Extra tubes are available as are filters designed to restrict moisture from entering the tone generator.

2. Servox Inton

This device, manufactured by Siemens, is an electronic, neck-held sound source that is easily adapted for oral use as well. An adapter is simply placed over the head of the instrument, and an oral tube is inserted into the opening. The unit is tubular and sealed in a scratch resistant case (Figure 4–4). It is fairly lightweight, offers volume and pitch control, and features rechargeable batteries. The recharger (Figure 4–4) is included in the cost

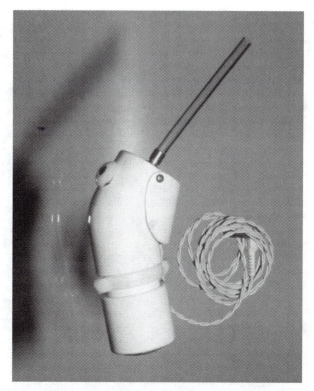

Figure 4–3. Extended grip tone generator for the Cooper-Rand. (Photo courtesy of Luminaud.)

of the complete kit and can charge two batteries simultaneously. The Servox Inton has a wide frequency range and is durable. The battery is reported to hold a charge for 7 hours.

3. Romet Speech-Aid

This device, manufactured by Romet, is a small, lightweight (5 oz), neck-held electronic sound source that uses rechargeable batteries. The unit is held against the neck, a button is depressed to turn it on, and the sound is articulated by the patient. The unit is equipped with a volume control as well as a pitch control.

4. SPKR

This device, a product of UNI Manufacturing Company, is another electronic, hand-held sound source that is placed

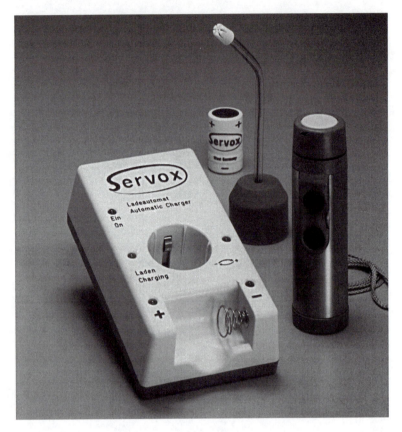

Figure 4–4. The Servox Inton electronic speech aid, oral adapter, battery, and charger unit. (Photo courtesy of Siemans Corporation.)

against the neck to direct sound through the skin into the vocal tract. It features a dual tone rocker switch, a volume control, an external pitch adjustment, and an oral adapter. It uses recharge-able batteries and has a safety strap.

5. Denrick Speech Aid

This instrument (Figure 4–5) has a unique rectangular shape and is relatively small. It features the option of internal Ni-Cad batteries, household current, or a 9-volt battery for operation. It has a built-in charger which restores the battery to 70% in less than 3 hours. An external recharger is also available. The Denrick has a variety of tones and is available in a variety of colors. It is designed as a neck-held unit.

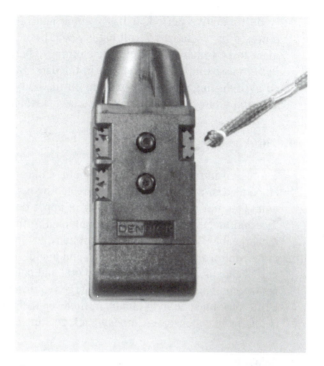

Figure 4–5. Denrick speech aid. (Photo courtesy of Luminaud.)

6. TruTone Electronic Speech Aid

Manufactured by Griffin Laboratories, this is a small, lightweight unit in a durable housing that operates on either rechargeable or regular 9-volt batteries. Volume is adjusted by turning the head of the instrument and pitch is varied using a pressure sensitive button. It comes with an oral adapter.

7. Nu-Vois Artificial Larynx

The Nu-Vois is designed as a neck-held unit but an intraoral adapter is included. It is lightweight and offers control of pitch and volume. It has a single switch operation and uses rechargeable 9-volt batteries. A recharging unit is provided.

8. P.O.Vox

The P.O.Vox is a lightweight, inexpensive, disposable, sterile, intraoral device that is designed for single-patient use in the early postoperative period. It has volume and pitch controls, is powered by a standard 9-volt battery, and has a clip for attachment to bed linens or articles of clothing. There is a flashing light to assist in locating the unit in the dark. Sound is activated by light finger or hand pressure on the body of the device. The oral tubing has an endpiece that is removable for cleaning.

9. UltraVoice

This is an intraoral device from Health Concepts, Inc. that is embedded in a dental plate and activated by a small hand-held unit. The oral unit is mounted into an upper denture or an orthodontic retainer. The batteries contained in this oral unit are rechargeable. The hand-held control activates the sound by remote control and also controls pitch and loudness. The charging unit is capable of charging both the oral and hand-held components simultaneously with a full charge requiring 8 hours. The UltraVoice must be individually crafted for each individual and is relatively expensive. A money back guarantee is offered.

10. SolaTone

This new neck-held instrument is light and compact and has a single tone button. It operates on a 9-volt battery and has both pitch and volume adjustments. It is reported to be very durable. It may be more economical than other similar instruments.

11. Optivox Electrolarynx

Bivona, Inc. has recently introduced the Optivox Electrolarynx. It is slightly larger and heavier than some of the other units but has several unique features. The Optivox pitch adjustment is located internally but in an easily accessible manner and requires no tools for adjustment. A small dial is easily moved to set the desired pitch level which then remains constant. The volume dial is external. The outer sleeve is made of impact resistant aluminum which is available in several colors. The manufacturers cite tonal purity and clarity which do not depend on any adjustments of the sounding head. It works with all 9-volt style batteries, and the complete kit contains an oral connector and tubes.

C. Advantages

The major advantage of the electric-powered speech aids (and to some degree the pneumatic devices) is the ability to offer a rapidly learned means of communication. The devices can be demonstrated prior to surgery and require little effort to use immediately after surgery. They are easily portable. Some permit a limited ability to vary the fundamental frequency of the voice during speech to achieve some measure of pitch inflection. Many are available with an intraoral adapter. The adapter fits over the membrane or vibrator and usually uses a small plastic tube to direct the sound into the vocal tract. This adapter permits the use of the instrument immediately after surgery when the neck wound is healing. Patients experience an immediate restoration of their ability to communicate. After wound healing is complete, patients may have the option of using the device in either manner, for example, against the skin of the neck or as an oral unit, depending on which placement provides optimally intelligible speech.

D. Disadvantages

All of these devices tend to produce a mechanical sound that may be distracting to a listener and may interfere with communication. Most require the use of one hand, limiting the ability of the patient to use both hands when talking. Most have very limited control of fundamental frequency, which limits normal pitch inflection of the patient's speech. In addition, it may be cumbersome to use the pitch-altering mechanisms that are available. There are some operating expenses, because the batteries wear out, and mechanical devices may need occasional repair.

E. Indications for Use

1. An **oral** type of instrument can be used effectively soon after surgery, regardless of the type of alaryngeal speech the patient will choose to pursue, including those who expect to pursue tracheoesophageal speech.

2. **Electronic speech aids** are a helpful adjunct for persons learning esophageal speech. They can be used for communication, thereby reducing the frustrations of speechlessness.

3. An electronic speech aid may be a **preferred primary means of communication** for some persons. Patients who are elderly and infirm and whose life-style involves minimal communication may choose an instrument.

4. A person who is very **eager to speak** and cannot tolerate the frustration or demands for practicing esophageal speech may be happy with an instrument.

5. The person who **cannot master esophageal speech** and does not wish to undergo further surgery may choose to use an electronic instrument.

6. All **laryngectomees** should have an instrument and know how to use it as a backup or insurance policy in case of emergency or other situations when other forms of alaryngeal speech may fail or be inadequate.

III. ESOPHAGEAL SPEECH

A. Description

Esophageal speech involves the production of a voice source within the esophagus using air supplied by the patient. The esophagus is a muscular tube that begins just behind the larynx. The most inferior portion of the inferior constrictor muscle, called the cricopharyngeus, extends from the cricoid cartilage to insert on portions of the pharynx posteriorly and into the esophagus. Surgeons attempt to leave this muscle intact during laryngectomy, so it can be used to constrict the esophagus and permit the trapping of air inferiorly. When the air is expelled through a narrow constriction in the esophagus created by the cricopharyngeus muscle, the narrowed segment (the pharyngoesophageal or PE segment) will vibrate, producing sound.

B. Anatomy of Esophageal Speech

1. Surgical Alterations

Surgery for laryngeal carcinoma may involve only the larynx (and associated extrinsic muscles), or it may require the extirpation of other structures and muscles in the neck. Consequently, the exact anatomical changes that a patient may experience depend on the extent of the carcinoma and the surgical requirements for its complete excision. However, most surgeons will attempt to salvage as much anatomy as is safely possible.

In the simplest case, the patient may have lost only the larynx. This means, of course, that the source of sound for speech is missing. The larynx and the hyoid bone are typically removed during a routine laryngectomy. The trachea is sutured to the front of the neck where a permanent opening called the tracheostoma is created. These changes are illustrated in Figure 4–6. On the left are the normal anatomical relationships among the larynx, esophagus, pharynx, and oral and nasal cavities. On the right are the surgical alterations to this anatomy that result from a laryngectomy. There are, of course, little or no surgical changes to the esophagus during the procedure. However, esophageal speech depends on the ability of the esophagus to constrict at about the region shown by the dotted lines in the figure. This region is known as the pharyngoesophageal segment (or simply the PE segment).

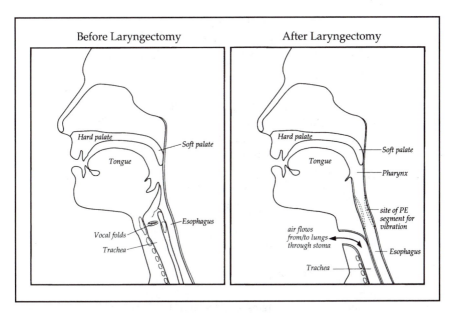

Figure 4–6. Schematic of the anatomy of the head and neck prior to (left panel) and after (right panel) laryngectomy.

2. PE Segment

This refers to that portion of the pharynx and esophagus where muscle fibers from the inferior constrictor, cricopharyngeus (or the lower portion of the inferior constrictor), and the esophagus blend together (see Figure 4–7). This creates a potential sphincter that can decrease the cross-sectional area of the esophagus. Although most of the esophagus is composed of muscle fibers not under voluntary control, the muscle fibers in the upper portion of the esophagus are under voluntary control. Thus, an individual can exert conscious control of the upper esophagus. The criopharyngeus muscle extends posteriorly from the cricoid car-

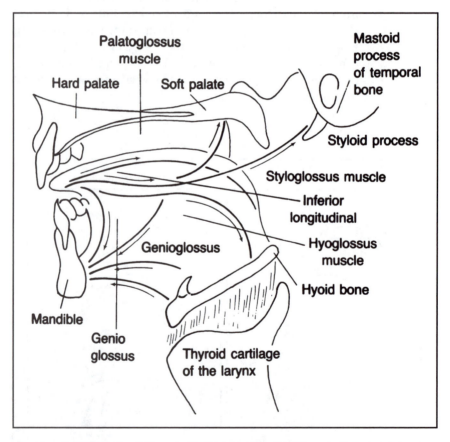

Figure 4–7. Schematic of the muscles of the tongue and pharynx. (From Zemlin, W., Speech and Hearing Science. [3rd ed.]. Englewood Cliffs NJ: Prentice-Hall, 1988. Copyright 1988 by Prentice-Hall. Reprinted by permission.)

tilage of the larynx and blends with the muscle fibers of the esophagus. During laryngectomy surgery, the anterior fibers of the cricopharyngeus are sutured together, creating a complete muscle sphincter around the esophagus. The shape and length of the PE segment varies depending on the exact surgical alterations to the anatomy of the region. However, shape or size of the PE segment do appear to be factors in predicting successful acquisition of esophageal speech. Of even greater importance is the degree of tonicity of the segment. If the resistance of the PE segment to dilation or oscillation is high, it may be difficult for the patient to insufflate the esophagus to produce good esophageal vibrations.

3. Air Supply

Esophageal speakers have a much lower air reservoir (less than 100 cc) than is available to laryngeal speakers from the lungs (>5 liters). However, this small air supply need not be a significant limitation to good sound production. Efficient esophageal speakers, as well as laryngeal speakers, typically require a very small amount of air to produce vibration. The small air supply will limit the esophageal speaker's ability to produce long utterances on a single charge of air.

Air flow rates are also somewhat variable in esophageal speakers and depend on the volume of air in the esophagus, the pressure within the esophagus, and the resistance of the PE segment (Diedrich, 1991).

4. Air Discharge

Air is thought to be expelled from the esophagus as a result of mechanisms similar to exhalation of air from the lungs. That is, increased thoracic pressure creates a force on the esophagus (which passes through the thorax on its way to the stomach). The esophageal walls within the thorax are constricted, forcing the air within to move up the esophagus and out the mouth. Interestingly, there is evidence (Kahrilas et al., 1986) that in laryngeal speakers, during a belch, the pressure in the upper portion of the esophagus is lower than in the lower portion of the esophagus. This suggests that the resistance to opening the upper portion of the esophagus is less than the lower portion, permitting easier egress of air upward into the pharynx rather than downward into the stomach. It is not known if similar relationships exist in the laryngectomized individual, but if they do, it could help explain why pressures in the thorax force air upward into the pharynx rather than downward into the stomach.

C. Techniques for Obtaining an Air Supply

1. Injection

In this method, air is injected from the mouth into the esophagus via the tongue and pharynx. The tongue acts like a piston to force air back into the pharynx and esophagus. There are two stages in this sequence. First, the tongue pushes air in the mouth back to the pharynx (the so-called glossal press). Second, the back of the tongue and pharynx force the air down into the esophagus. These movements must be coordinated smoothly. There are two major variations of this process, one depends on the extent of surgery and the structures remaining intact, and the other depends on the patient's ability to master the technique. Diedrich and Youngstrom (1966; Trudeau & Qi, 1990) described these maneuvers in their classic study of alaryngeal speech.

a. The **glossal press** is produced by the tongue tip contacting the alveolar ridge. The midportion of the tongue may elevate to contact the hard palate. Air is trapped behind the tongue and moved posteriorly by the backward movement of the tongue. The tongue does not make actual contact with the posterior pharyngeal wall. However, the soft palate is elevated to prevent escape of the air through the nose. The lips may or may not be closed because the tongue tip traps the air needed for injection.

b. In the **glossopharyngeal press**, tongue movement is similar to that seen in the glossal press, but the tongue continues to move backward to contact the pharyngeal wall. Again, velopharyngeal closure is necessary, but lip closure is not.

Some patients may feel the need to close their lips for this maneuver and may add buccal movements in the attempt to push the air back. These are not necessary and should be eliminated as the patient achieves mastery of the technique. Other patients may trap air in the pharynx and produce pharyngeal (Donald Duck) speech. For obvious reasons, this type of sound production should be avoided.

2. Inhalation Method

In this method, the patient must lower the pressure within the esophageal segment relative to the atmospheric pressure. This permits air to flow from the outside (or inside the mouth) to the lower than normal pressure area in the esophagus. To accomplish this, the patient must be able to relax the PE segment, otherwise, air cannot flow downward. Typically, the intraesophageal pressure is between −4 and −15 mm Hg below atmospheric pressure (Diedrich, 1991). When the PE segment opens, air in the mouth and pharynx which is typically at atmospheric pressure (+14 mm Hg) will naturally flow from the region of higher pressure to the region of lower pressure in the esophagus. The reduction of pressure within the esophagus is a by-product of the normal inhalation of pulmonary air. That is, when the speaker inhales air, the pressure within the esophagus becomes even more negative relative to the atmosphere (as much as −15 mm Hg), creating an even greater sucking force to pull the air into the esophagus. The forces that are responsible for the inhalation (and exhalation) of air within the thorax also help in the "inhalation" (and exhalation) of air from the esophagus.

3. Swallowing

At one time or another, each of us has swallowed air into the stomach and has, at a later time, burped. But, swallowing air is not advantageous for creating an air supply for esophageal speech for a variety of reasons.

a. Swallowing is a reflex that requires a bolus of some type to trigger the reflex action. In the absence of a trigger, it is often difficult to initiate a swallow.

b. It is not possible to "dry swallow" quickly and repetitively as required for speech.

c. Voluntary control of the air supply from the stomach may be very difficult to achieve, if not impossible.

D. Advantages

Esophageal speech may offer a number of advantages over other forms of communication.

1. There are no external, visually distracting devices necessary.

2. The sound of esophageal speech is more "natural" and nearly like that produced by the vocal folds (although usually of much lower fundamental frequency).

3. The patient is able to achieve some measure of pitch and loudness control, and good esophageal speakers are able to vary these dynamically during speech.

4. There are no batteries that run down or devices that break down.

5. Both hands are free during the speech act.

E. Disadvantages

1. Esophageal speech must be learned and may take a long time to master. Some patients may never learn to produce functional esophageal speech even after much effort. Others may become frustrated during the learning process.

2. A person's ability to articulate clearly must be excellent, otherwise the intelligibility of esophageal speech may be poor.

3. The patient may have difficulty being heard above background noise. There are speech amplifiers available from various manufacturers (Voicette, Rand Voice Amplifier, Personal Talker Voice Amplifier, Flex-Mike, AddVox, or Mini-Vox) (see Appendix D) that can be used to increase loudness.

4. There is some experimental evidence that suggests listeners find esophageal speech least preferable in comparison to other types of alternative sound production (Carpenter, 1991). However, there is other evidence that suggests esophageal speech is preferred to speech produced with electronic or pneumatic speech aids.

F. Indications for Use of Esophageal Speech

1. Most patients are potential esophageal speakers. The exceptions to this might be patients with extensive pharyngeal, esophageal, lingual, and/or mandibular resection; patients whose medical status is otherwise compromised; patients with significant hearing loss; patients who have chosen to have surgical prosthetic voice restoration; and patients who have no desire to learn esophageal speech.

2. Patients can use esophageal speech and electronic speech aids interchangeably, depending on the environmental noise level or situation.

IV. TRACHEOESOPHAGEAL PUNCTURE (TEP)

A. Description

Tracheoesophageal puncture is a surgical, endoscopic voice restoration procedure in which a small puncture is made through the tracheoesophageal party wall into the esophagus. This provides a conduit for pulmonary air to drive the vibration of the pharyngoesophageal vibratory segment to create sound. The sound travels into the pharynx, then into the oral and nasal cavities where it is resonated and articulated to produce speech (Figure 4–8). A prosthesis that contains a one-way valve is placed into the tract to prevent aspiration, maintain the patency of the puncture, and allow the flow of air into the esophagus for voice production. Examples of the prostheses used in this procedure are shown in Figures 4–9 and 4–10.

B. Description of Surgical Procedure

Tracheoesophageal puncture may be performed at the time of laryngectomy (primary puncture) or may be performed postoperatively after sufficient healing has occurred (secondary puncture). Primary puncture is usually reserved for uncomplicated cases of total laryngectomy in which extended pharyngeal or esophageal reconstruction is not required. Secondary puncture is usually delayed a minimum of 6 weeks after the completion of postoperative radiation therapy, or if combined therapies, for example, surgery and radiation, are not required, 6 weeks postlaryngectomy. Maintaining the surgically created puncture until it has healed is accomplished by placing a catheter (or in the case of a primary puncture, the feeding tube) through the puncture site downward into the esophagus. The catheter is subsequently removed by the surgeon or speech-language pathologist when the voice prosthesis is fitted.

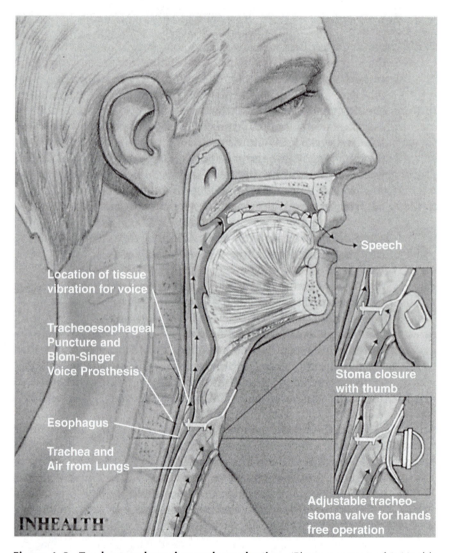

Figure 4–8. Tracheoesophageal speech production. (Photo courtesy of InHealth Corporation.)

C. Voice Prosthesis

The voice prosthesis is a short (1.4–3.6 cm) tube of medically safe material (usually silicone) with a one-way valve (slit, hinge, or ball type) at the distal portion. The anterior, or front, end has an opening through which pulmonary air enters the prosthesis. The distal end is inserted into the esophagus and has a small collar (or flange)

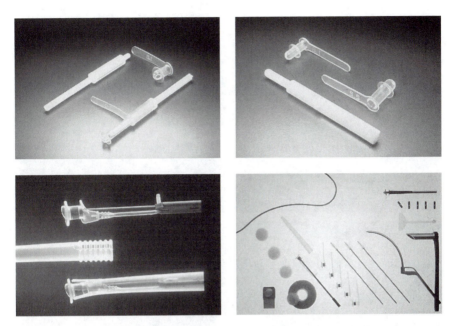

Figure 4–9. Tracheoesophageal puncture prostheses available from Bivona Corporation. Upper left panel: low resistance voice prosthesis with insertion tool (bottom of picture). Upper Right Panel: Duckbill voice prosthesis, Lower Left Panel: Provox 2 indwelling voice prosthesis, Lower Right Panel: Provox voice restoration system. (Photo courtesy of Bivona Corporation.)

to aid in retention of the prosthesis. The diameter of the prosthesis is typically French 16 or French 20.

The earliest prostheses developed by Singer and Blom were of the duckbill type, with approximately 8 mm of the distal tip extending into the esophagus. Prosthesis sizes were established by measuring the length of the prosthesis from the distal tip to the tracheal flange or strap. Later designs typically have a shorter distal tip or may only have a retention collar that protrudes into the esophagus. American manufacturers had initially sized these prostheses to maintain a comparable interflange distance relative to the corresponding duckbill prosthesis without regard for the overall length. Thus, a size 2.2 low pressure voice prosthesis would have the same interflange length as a 2.2 duckbill prosthesis, despite the fact that the overall length of the low pressure prosthesis is shorter, owing to its reduced distal tip. More recently, American and European manufacturers have attempted to standardize prosthesis sizing by specifying only the interflange length of the prosthesis in millimeters.

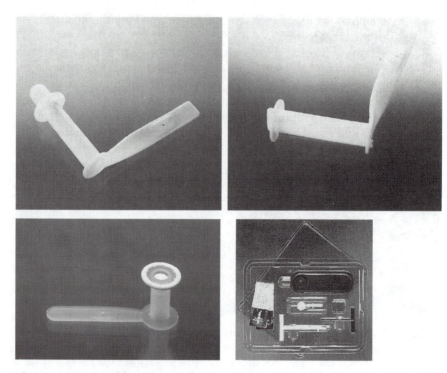

Figure 4–10. InHealth voice prosthesis and accessories. Upper Left Panel: Duckbill voice prosthesis, Upper Right Panel: Low pressure voice prosthesis, Lower Left Panel: Indwelling voice prosthesis, Lower Right Panel: Indwelling kit. (Photos courtesy of InHealth Corporation.)

Air pressures required to open the prosthesis valve typically vary between 2 and 100 cm H_2O and depend on the rate of airflow from the lungs and the type of device employed (Heaton, Sanderson, Dunsmore, & Parker, 1996; Weinberg & Moon, 1984). Lower opening pressures, allowing for greater ease of sound production, characterize many of the more recent prosthesis designs. These "low resistance" prostheses incorporate hinge- or ball-type valves that open with less respiratory effort or they have a larger diameter (20 French), which allows greater airflow through the prosthesis than the original duckbill model. The reader is referred to the prosthetic manufacturers for aerodynamic specifications of the various devices that are currently available.

D. Mechanisms of TEP Sound Production

1. To produce sound with the voice prosthesis in place, the patient uses his or her own air supply from the lungs. To do so, the patient inhales, then occludes the stoma with a finger or thumb, and exhales. Air from the lungs enters the lumen of the prosthesis, opens the one-way valve, and is released into the esophagus. This air passes through the PE segment, setting it into vibration to generate sound (see Figure 4–8).

2. The sound produced enters the oral cavity where it is articulated and shaped into words. With practice, the laryngectomee learns to produce complete sentences with normal rate and phrasing.

3. The patient quickly learns to **coordinate stomal occlusion and release** to meet the alternating respiratory and phonatory requirements. Special tracheostoma valves are also available which eliminate manual occlusion of the stoma, resulting in hands-free speech and added hygenic benefits. These valves close automatically when greater than normal thoracic pressures are present as when, for example, the patient wishes to produce speech, but return to an open position as pressures are reduced to allow quiet respiration.

E. Advantages

This technique can provide the most rapid restoration of near normal speech for most laryngectomized patients. Appropriate selection criteria need to be employed (see Chapter 6). After sufficient healing has occurred, the prosthesis can be fitted easily by the physician/ speech pathologist team. After appropriate instruction, most patients learn to remove and reinsert the device and perform the necessary maintenance. Extended wear prostheses (InHealth® Indwelling, Provox®, Groningen, Voice Master®) require minimal maintenance by the laryngectomee and infrequent replacements (approximately every 4 to 6 months) by the physician or speech-language pathologist. Prostheses are available in a variety of sizes and styles to accommodate variations in tracheoesophageal wall thickness and individual aerodynamic requirements for speech production. The use of a tracheostomal valve enables hands-free speech.

The other major advantage is that pulmonary air is used to drive the vibration of the PE segment, permitting ample air supply for the production of utterances of normal length and freeing the artic-ulators from the highly complex maneuvers of esophageal air intake. Experience with surgical prosthetic voice restoration has demonstrated a very high success rate (85–95%) in the acquisition of intelligible speech (Maniglia, Lundy, Casiano & Swiontkowski, 1989; McEwan et al., 1996).

F. Disadvantages

1. As with any surgery, there are risks, albeit small. The possibili-ty of complications that may compromise the airway or punc-ture is present.

2. Occasionally, the puncture may stenose, preventing the insertion of the device and resulting in loss of voice. This usually occurs if the puncture has been allowed to remain totally unstented or if the prosthesis has been fitted incorrectly (undersized).

3. There is a slight risk of aspiration of the prosthesis if it becomes dislodged from its correct placement.

4. Other reported complications include stoma stenosis, radiation-induced closure of the puncture, granulation tissue build-up, prolapse, or leakage around the prosthesis with subsequent aspi-ration of saliva or liquids.

5. The patient is dependent on the prosthesis to maintain the punc-ture and prevent aspiration. The laryngectomee must be respon-sible for routine maintenance and must develop an understand-ing of the function of the prosthesis.

V. SUMMARY

Various alaryngeal speech modes are available so that no laryngec-tomee should be without a means of communication. There are a vari-ety of artificial devices that can be used to produce a source of sound, including those that use the patient's own air to drive a sound source and electronic devices that produce a battery driven sound. Alternatively, the patient can learn a new form of voicing using a muscular segment of the esophagus as a source of sound. Surgically, a puncture can be created through the tracheoesophageal wall, a prothesis placed in it to divert pulmonary air into the esophagus, and using that same muscular segment, sound is produced. Some of these sound source alternatives may be used immediately after surgery to restore voice, whereas others are delayed and require a period of learning. Many factors enter into the choice of which alternative to use with a particular patient. These are discussed further in Chapters 5 and 6.

CHAPTER

5

Teaching Alaryngeal Speech

Various aspects of the rehabilitation process were discussed in Chapter 3. They are germane to the topic of this chapter as well and are in many ways inseparable from what happens during the therapeutic process. In Chapter 4, the various modes of alaryngeal speech were described along with the indications for choosing each. In some instances, that choice will be made in consultation with the surgeon prior to the laryngectomy, whereas in others, the choice is left to the patient. The speech-language pathologist plays a role in helping the patient make an informed choice by providing objective information and allowing the patient a trial period of instrument use and esophageal speech instruction. The need for a surgical puncture procedure precludes a trial of tracheoesophageal (TEP) speech. The primary goal of rehabilitation is functional communication, regardless of the method selected.

In this chapter, we begin with a discussion of some general considerations that apply to laryngectomee rehabilitation regardless of the mode of speech that will be pursued. The remainder of the chapter is devoted to discussion of teaching techniques for the use of pneumatic and electronic speech aids and for developing esophageal speech. (Chapter 6 is devoted to discussion of all aspects of the TEP.)

The absence of a specific section on assessment or evaluation should not be considered an oversight. Because the speech-language pathologist often has several contacts with a patient prior to the initiation of "formal" speech treatment, those contacts generally form the basis of an ongoing evaluation. In earlier chapters, we stressed the need for the speech-language pathologist to be knowledgeable about the nature and extent of the surgery and other treatment that the patient has had or is having. That information forms part of the assessment. In Chapter 3, numerous prognostic factors and areas of concern were discussed. These must be considered by the speech-language pathologist as part of the assessment process to ensure appropriate testing is done and referrals made.

I. GENERAL CONSIDERATIONS

A few broad areas apply to all alaryngeal speech modes, although some may be most relevant to one or another of the speech modes. These include initiation of therapy, group versus individual therapy, frequency of therapy, involvement of family and/or friends in the therapy session, practice and pace of therapy, prognostic factors, and when to terminate therapy. Issues of reimbursement are too complex and changeable to be discussed here.

A. Timing of Speech Therapy

1. We advocate the **earliest possible initiation of speech therapy**. All patients have the right to some viable form of communication in the shortest time possible as long as it does not interfere with or jeopardize their recovery from surgery or their medical condition. Often therapy may start during the preoperative period or the inpatient hospital stay. If not, patients are strongly encouraged to begin speech therapy as soon after discharge from the hospital as possible, assuming that medical clearance has been obtained from the surgeon. It is important to begin the rehabilitation process promptly because the longer the time between the surgery and the beginning of therapy, the poorer the prospects for a good result. Many patients will have to undergo a course of radiation therapy postoperatively; a difficult period often lasting 5 to 7 weeks. Many have physical re-

actions to the radiation treatment that may retard or interrupt the process of speech acquisition. It is important for the new laryngectomee to have acquired some form of communication (other than writing) prior to radiation. Furthermore, lack of involvement in the rehabilitation process for a period of 1 to 2 months (or more), particularly in the absence of a viable means of communication, can lead to feelings of isolation, depression, and frustration.

a. **Patients are usually ready to begin esophageal speech training** shortly after they begin to take food by mouth. The beginning of oral feeding suggests that wound healing has progressed to the point where attempts to produce sound will not jeopardize further recovery.

b. **Use of an oral type of electronic speech aid can often begin within days after laryngectomy surgery**, assuming the patient's recovery is without complications. The extent of the lesion and of the surgery must be considered when judging the patient's readiness for using an electronic speech aid.

c. **Use of a neck-held electronic speech aid can begin as soon as healing of the surgical suture lines is complete and swelling has resolved** sufficiently to obtain good transcutaneous transmission of sound.

d. In the case of TEP, **readiness for initiation of speech with a prosthesis** depends on the healing of the puncture site. Additionally, in the case of primary puncture, healing of the esophagus and neck tissues should be sufficient to the degree that the patient has resumed an oral diet.

2. **Early use of a speech aid** can decrease feelings of isolation, depression, and frustration. In uncomplicated cases, an oral type of electronic speech aid can be introduced a few days postsurgically along with instruction in its use. In the first days following surgery patients may not feel well enough to put forth the necessary effort to learn a new way of speaking. If the patient's initial attempts with an electronic speech aid are not completely successful, further attempts are made on subsequent days, with reassurance that this is not necessarily a prediction of future failure with the instrument. In some cases it may be desirable to wait until the patient is discharged from the hospital.

B. Group Versus Individual Therapy

Each approach has its advantages and disadvantages and may be determined by the type of alaryngeal speech to be pursued, patient preference, clinician style, and scheduling constraints. The fitting of a prosthesis is best done individually, as is the initial instruction in producing tracheoesophageal speech. For those patients who will pursue either esophageal speech training or the use of an electronic speech aid, or both, the choice of group versus individual therapy can be considered.

1. **Individual therapy,** of course, provides the patient with the full and undivided attention of the speech-language pathologist. The amount of time given directly to the individual patient is greater than can be provided to any one individual in a group setting. Some patients become anxious and self-conscious in the presence of a group and may not learn as fast or as well as when alone.

2. **Group therapy,** on the other hand, exposes the individual to others who "are in the same boat" thus lessening the feelings of isolation. It allows for interchange among group members about shared concerns other than speech. Newly laryngectomized persons benefit from the models presented by others in the group who are farther along in the process. The group approach relieves some of the pressure on any one individual by spreading the time across all group members. Members of the group provide support and encouragement for each other. It is true, of course, that those in the group who are slower to acquire esophageal speech may observe others learn more quickly and "graduate," while they are still making slow progress. This can be a source of some frustration, but it can be used in positive ways. Handling a group therapy session is perhaps more challenging for the speech-language pathologist than individual therapy. When patients are at different stages of learning it is necessary to address each one's needs without losing the rest of the group or wasting their time. Often there will be a patient who attempts to monopolize much of the time and the clinician is challenged to work around that behavior without alienating that patient. The group experience is so helpful to most patients that, despite the difficulties, we encourage all clinicians who work with laryngectomees to try it. Frequently, a patient who has been successful and whose formal therapy has ended will continue to come to group sessions. These patients serve as role

models and sources of support for other members of the group. They also derive benefit from this experience, thus, everyone benefits.

a. **Methods of structuring a group therapy session** will differ based on the composition of the group. The following are general methods that we have found to be effective.

   (1) **Each session lasts 90 minutes.** For small groups of two to four people, 60 minutes may be adequate.

   (2) **Introduction and general conversation** may take up to 10 minutes. This usually involves greeting each person and finding out how the week has gone for each individual. Comments that are made during this time may elicit some useful group discussion. It is important to keep this structured so that it does not take an inordinate proportion of the therapy time.

   (3) **A brief "warm-up" period** may follow during which everyone is encouraged to produce esophageal sound, if they can, or tracheoesophageal sound. This is done as a group giving the patients a chance to produce sound without being the direct object of everyone's focus.

   (4) **Each person, in turn, then receives individual attention.** This time is addressed to the specific goal(s) being worked on by each individual. Feedback and assistance are offered. When a patient is observed to be reinforcing a mistake by repeated practice of an incorrect production or act, this is noted and brought to the patient's attention. An effort is made to correct the mistake. If the patient is unable to change the behavior, it may be necessary to revert to practicing an earlier level task. If the patient is ready to move to another goal it is introduced during this time. While the clinician's attention is focused on one individual, others in the group may be encouraged to continue practicing a task. This requires that the clinician be able to split attention so that feedback or encouragement can be given when a patient does some task well.

   (5) If the group contains both very advanced speakers and beginning speakers, **it can be helpful to create subgroups** for a part of the session. The advanced speakers can help each other while the clinician focuses on the beginning group. Pairing an advanced speaker with a beginning speaker can also be effective. Advanced speakers may be called on to present stimulus items to the rest of the group under the direction of the clinician. This

provides a challenge for the advanced speaker, thus serving the needs of both groups.

(6) At the end of the session, **each person's practice assignment for the coming week is discussed**. It is important for the clinician to be specific in giving assignments, including what is to be done, how it is to be done, how often, and for how long. Written instructions are helpful.

3. A **combined approach** offers the best of both individual and group therapy. Patients can be seen individually for the first part of their initial outpatient visit. This allows the speech-language pathologist to determine how the patient is doing, to explore which model of electronic instrument will provide the best speech possible for the person, to begin instruction in that mode of speech if it has not been begun before, and to introduce production of esophageal sound. Patients can then be introduced into the group class with the understanding that the option to choose individual sessions is available. And conversely, the clinician may feel that a patient in the group would benefit from additional attention and can suggest supplementary individual therapy on an as-needed basis. Sometimes one or two individual sessions during a particularly difficult point in therapy can help the patient progress to the next level. Most patients are anxious to continue with the group classes as well.

C. Frequency of Therapy Sessions

There are no hard and fast rules about the frequency patients should be seen. Once again, the type of alaryngeal speech the patient will pursue must be considered in discussion of therapeutic needs.

1. The **frequency of visits for the laryngectomee pursuing tracheoesophageal speech** will be determined by the patient's need, the clinician's philosophy and time constraints, and the availability of funding.

   a. In the case of secondary TEP, the first visit ideally occurs prior to surgery. At this time, the speech pathologist (in conjunction with the physician) assesses the various factors that may influence **candidacy** for undergoing the surgical procedure. These include the vibratory capabilities of the PE segment (see section on esophageal insufflation testing), articulation, manual dexterity, adequacy of vision, and cognitive potential for comprehending the use of the device. This also provides the opportunity to present basic information regarding the method of tracheoesophageal voice restoration using anatomy diagrams, printed materials, and prosthesis models. It is often helpful to show videotaped examples of tracheoesophageal speakers so that the patient and caregiver have realistic expectations regarding the postsurgical outcomes.

b. In the **case of primary TEP**, the speech pathologist should have had the opportunity to begin discussion concerning the method of prosthetic voice restoration during the postoperative hospitalization period.

c. In either primary or secondary TEP, **visits begin** with the fitting of the voice prosthesis. Additional visits and their timing will depend on the initial success with the prosthesis and the patient's learning how to use and maintain the device (see Chapter 6).

d. Because the acquisition of esophageal speech usually takes longer than TEP speech, the question of **frequency of esophageal speech classes is critical**. Although a period of intensive daily or twice daily therapy might result in faster acquisition of esophageal speech, it is usually not a viable option due to physical stamina, distance to travel to the therapy site, scheduling of clinical time, and cost. Practically, it is best to see patients once a week. In general, this frequency of therapy sessions works well. It provides time for patients to practice a given skill and to reinforce previously learned skills, it is frequent enough without generating pressure, and it also provides a period of time during which the patient begins to adjust to the changes brought about by the surgery.

e. Frequency of visits for those who choose to use an electronic speech aid can also be once a week. Indeed, the group situation may encompass people using two or even three modes of speech. Overall duration of therapy for those patients choosing to use an electronic speech aid as their primary mode of communication will usually be shorter than for acquisition of esophageal speech. Patients can benefit from practice time between sessions, and they have additional time to adjust to their new circumstance.

D. Involvement of Family and/or Friends in Therapy Sessions

Involvement of significant others is always encouraged. It is especially important during the initial session, at the very least, so that family and/or friends can gain a basic understanding of the rehabilitation process and, specifically, speech rehabilitation. Of course, the amount of involvement must always be tempered by sensitivity to the relationship between the persons involved. Supportive family members or close friends can be a major source of help for the patient and can be more effective when they understand the process. The opposite is also true. That is, the family member or friend who may be experiencing difficulty accepting the changes in the laryngectomee may react in ways that may be harmful and destructive. Of course, if the relationship was a troubled one prior to the surgery, those troubles will persist, and will probably be aggravated. It is often helpful to invite accompanying persons to attend the therapy sessions when they choose to do so. This type of open invitation allows those who are interested to be observers while not putting pressure on those who do not care to observe. Rarely does a spouse or other family member or friend observe every time. Most will observe for one or two sessions and then may prefer to spend time in the waiting room talking with those who have accompanied other patients. That too, may be therapeutic.

E. Pace of Therapy and Practice

1. The pace of therapy with the patient using a tracheoesophageal prosthesis is not problematic. As healing of the puncture site occurs, the clinician selects the prosthetic device that will enable the best quality speech and meet other requirements for ease of insertion, retention, and durability. When the patient gains the ability to produce sound and speech easily and understands the potential complications and the techniques of device maintenance, he or she is usually able to progress rapidly and gain skill with experience.

2. Similarly, the pace of therapy for electronic speech aid use is straightforward. After the patient has mastered the ability to produce speech, additional training in improving clarity of articulation and management of rate of speech, if needed, is uncomplicated.

3. The pace of esophageal speech training can be a critical factor in its acquisition. It must be neither too fast nor too slow. The

temptation to proceed too rapidly is present for both the patient and the clinician. A few patients acquire esophageal speech production very quickly. It is, of course, necessary to allow progress to be as rapid as the patient can handle as long as the skill is being properly learned. Too often patients will attempt to converse when their skill with esophageal speech production has not attained that level of proficiency. This results in intermittent sound production, increased use of force and stoma blasting, and unintelligible speech. Patients must acquire the basic skill of easy, consistent, and rapid production of repetitive esophageal sound before they are truly able to converse in that mode. Training the musculature involved in this highly complex and coordinated act takes time and each step must be well established before proceeding to the next level of difficulty. Patients must be encouraged to use the electronic speech aid for general conversation until they have gained adequate skill to converse using esophageal speech.

F. Practice

Practice is essential for the development of all types of alaryngeal speech. However, the practice must be good practice. That is, the patient must understand not only what is to be practiced, but also how it is to be practiced, to be able through feedback to self-monitor the quality of what is being practiced, and to understand how long and how often the practice should be. Unless a patient demonstrates an understanding of a task and can assess when it is being done correctly, that task should not be assigned for home practice. Patients often practice incorrectly and adopt habits that can be difficult to change.

1. Written practice assignments are helpful. These should be prepared for each patient and should be explained clearly. Key words that have been used in the therapy session should be included to remind the patient of the goal of the practice.

2. Short but frequent practice sessions are most productive. Patients are instructed to practice for 5 to 10 minutes out of each half hour or hour. Short practice sessions tend to reduce frustration that may mount during longer sessions. Frequent practice makes it necessary for the patient to trigger the appropriate neuromuscular coordination many times. Because getting esophageal sound production started is often what patients find most difficult, increased frequency of practice sessions provides increased frequency of practice of sound initiation. Furthermore, frequent practice focuses attention on speech throughout the day, and after each session there is usually some "spill over" or generalization of what is being practiced for a period of time immediately following the practice. And finally, during the early stages of acquiring esophageal speech, patients frequently complain about feelings of fullness, of excess gas buildup, and sometimes of discomfort or increased heartburn. These feelings are the result of air taken in which, if not successfully or completely expelled in the production of esophageal sound, moves down to the stomach. Short practice sessions reduce that problem and allow time for whatever air has been taken into the stomach to be expelled naturally.

G. Prognostic Factors

These factors were discussed in Chapter 3. There is no clear way to determine how quickly or how well functional alaryngeal communication will be acquired. A statement of prognosis is a well educated guess.

1. The prognosis for **tracheoesophageal speech** following the surgical voice restoration procedure is probably most easily and reliably determined. Because the learning time for tracheoesophageal speech is typically very short, it is possible to judge relatively quickly how well the patient will do. Only a small percentage of patients have difficulty in producing speech following tracheoesophageal puncture and require additional workup and treatment. Most of the common problems in acquiring tracheoesophageal speech can be resolved through the selection of a prosthesis with optimum aerodynamic features. Caution must be exercised in making the judgment too soon because the healing process may result in alterations of the vibratory characteristics of the PE segment. Reduction of postoperative or postradiation edema may take up to 6 months, resulting in significant improvement of voicing capability after initial failures. Stricture or stenosis may occur at any time postlaryngectomy and may have a negative effect on speech production even after an initially positive outcome. If this is suspected, the patient should consult the surgeon.

2. Prognosis for the patient who chooses to use an **electronic speech aid** for purposes of communication can also be assessed

with fairly good accuracy. As a person begins to use the instrument, the ability to articulate clearly and place the instrument appropriately is quite obvious.

3. Prognosis for the acquisition of **functional esophageal speech** is problematic because it involves the learning of new skills that are more difficult to acquire than for either of the other two methods. As noted in Chapter 3, factors such as viability of the pharyngoesophageal segment, time elapsed since surgery, age, extent of surgery, hearing acuity, and personality must be considered. Even taking all those factors into account, the most skilled and experienced clinician can still make early prognostic judgments that are later proven to be incorrect. It may be best to err on the side of giving the patient the benefit of the doubt as long as he or she is motivated and making the effort to learn.

H. Termination of Therapy

Termination of therapy by the clinician requires careful, informed decision making.

1. For **tracheoesophageal speakers**, therapy is usually short term. Two criteria must be met: the patient is using intelligible, fluent speech with minimal effort and the patient (or responsible caregiver) demonstrates an understanding of the use and maintenance of the voice prosthesis, potential complications, and emergency procedures. In addition to the initial training sessions held soon after the puncture is created, patients fitted with the extended-wear type prostheses will require periodic visits (every 4–6 months) for prosthesis replacement, because these devices can only be fitted by a physician or speech-language pathologist.

2. Persons using electronic speech aids do not typically require extensive periods of therapy, and the end of therapy is usually obvious. **When the patient is using fluent speech that is readily intelligible to the untrained ear, therapy should be terminated**. The patient should also demonstrate understanding of the care of the electronic instrument, battery changing, and routine cleaning. Patients may be seen for one or two follow-up visits weeks or months after termination of therapy, or at their request.

3. The decision to terminate esophageal speech therapy can be affected by various factors. As long as a patient is making demon-

strable progress toward the therapeutic goals, the case for continuing therapy can be made. However, the number of sessions allowed may often be determined by the insurance company policies. Speech-language pathologists must become strong advocates for their patients in obtaining needed services. Generally, esophageal speech therapy should be terminated when the person is able to converse using readily intelligible esophageal speech as the primary mode of communication in most situations. That person's speech will continue to improve with use. When, after an adequate trial period, a laryngectomee seems unable to produce esophageal sound and appropriate testing has been carried out to rule out a physical reason for that inability (see section IV.E.2.d. for problems in teaching esophageal speech later in this chapter), it may become necessary for the clinician to counsel the patient to pursue one of the other forms of alaryngeal speech. The services of the social worker can often be helpful in these instances. There may be psychosocial or personal problems present that are influencing the patient's therapeutic course.

I.   Speech Aids as Insurance

It is appropriate for all laryngectomees, regardless of the type of alaryngeal speech they will use, to have a **speech aid as an insurance policy**. Unpredictable emergency situations may arise that could render either esophageal speech or tracheoesophageal speech useless or inadequate. The availability of a speech aid and some proficiency in its use could be essential.

J.   Honest Assessment

Honest assessment of the patient's speech is important. The clinician should never pretend to understand when, in fact, an utterance is unintelligible. When counseling patients about their therapeutic course, gentle honesty is always best.

II. NONSPEECH NEEDS

A. Hygiene

It is essential that patients adopt **stringent practices of hygiene** regarding the cleanliness and care of the stoma.

1. Some type of **stoma covering** should be worn at all times. This not only protects the patient by preventing foreign objects from

entering the airway, but it also is a means of maintaining some moisture around the area. This can be done by dampening the actual stoma covering material or attaching a piece of moist gauze to the undersurface of the cover.

2. The **stoma must be kept clean** and crust free. Heavy crusting can obstruct the opening, becomes difficult to remove, and irritates the skin. In addition, cleanliness helps to guard against any infection in the area.

3. All **plugs of mucus** must be removed to prevent obstruction of the airway.

B. Heat/Moisture Exchangers (HME)

1. The upper respiratory passages normally **filter, humidify, and warm inhaled air**. A total laryngectomy creates changed anatomical relationships in which the upper airway is bypassed for purposes of respiration. Filtration is diminished and humidification via the upper airway is lost. It is this humidifaction which helps to maintain the normally thin viscosity of mucus and allows it to be transported outward by cilia of the epithelial cells. The loss of these functions results in thickened and increased mucus secretions and drying of the respiratory tract. The thick mucus cannot be as readily transported outwardly and the drying creates irritation and stimulates frequent coughing.

2. Filters work on the principle that, during exhalation, heat and moisture are absorbed by the filter and transferred back to the incoming air during inhalation.

3. These filters are said to reduce coughing, reduce mucus production, improve breathing, and improve speech. It is our experience that these reports are essentially true but that a period of adjustment is required. The patient must be willing to adapt gradually to the presence of a filter which initially may feel as if it is interfering with the ability to breathe. The speech-language pathologist should exercise judgment in selecting patients who would benefit from the use of a filter.

4. There are several commercially available heat moisture exchange filters (Stom-Vent™, Stom-Vent2™, Provox™ Stom-afilter, InHealth [Blom-Singer] HumidiFilter) (Figure 5–1) which are designed to replace heat and moisture to the inhaled air as they filter it (Appendix D).

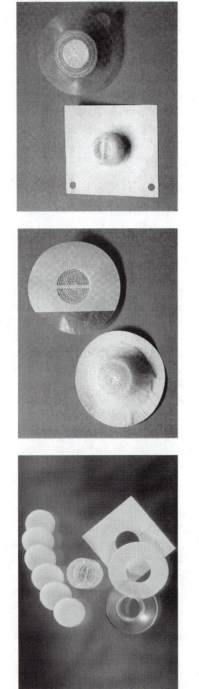

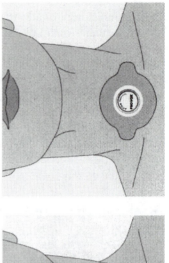

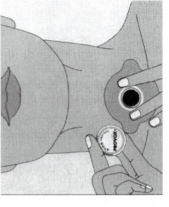

Figure 5–1. Heat moisture exchangers. Upper left panel: Humidifilter, Upper center panel: StomVent (Photo courtesy of Gibeck), Upper right panel: StomVent2 (Photo courtesy of Gibeck), Lower left panel: Provox Stoma filter with speech valve (Photo courtesy of Bivona), Lower right panel: Provox Stoma filter in place. (Photo courtesy of Bivona.)

a. The filters vary in design, airflow resistance, and efficiency. Their cost also varies. Grolman, Blom, Branson, Schouwenburg, and Hamaker (1997) have studied these factors for four specific HMEs and reported significant differences among them. None of the devices exceeded normal physiological upper airway resistance and although none attained what would be considered a perfect amount of moisture output, the StomVent 2 and the HumidiFilter rated the highest in moisture exchange. The HumidiFilter was found to be the least expensive.

b. The authors of this study stressed the need for considering the previous factors as well as factors of design and ease of use of the various HMEs when making recommendations for specific patients.

III. SPEECH AIDS

The comments that follow apply to the pneumatic and the electronic types of speech aids. It is generally accepted that speech aids serve a very useful purpose in providing most patients with a fairly rapidly learned means of communication that can free them from the tedium, frustration, and isolation of writing, or the limitations of whispering. Speech devices can be used as a short-term intermediate speech mode in anticipation of prosthetic voice restoration, as a temporary measure during the acquisition of esophageal speech, or as a viable and acceptable speech mode. The argument that these instruments are crutches and may deter a person's acquisition of another speech mode has not been demonstrated. Indeed, if a person breaks a leg, he or she will be happy to have a crutch. Its use will not impede healing and it may help the leg to heal more rapidly by restricting it from improper use.

A. Aid Selection

1. If the aid is to be **introduced soon after surgery**, it is appropriate to think about an instrument that can be placed in the mouth. A neck-held instrument should not be introduced until the suture lines have healed. Furthermore, it is necessary to consider any tenderness in the neck area and the presence of swelling. If swelling is present, transmission of sound transcutaneously will probably be poor.

2. If the aid is **introduced at a later stage**, following adequate healing, the patient should ideally be provided the opportunity to try various models of instruments to determine which one is best. (Recall that the intraoral device does not permit this type of trial, but should still be given consideration when appropriate.) The determination of "best" should be based primarily on the intelligibility of the speech produced. The clinician must offer guidance and feedback about this. Persons accompanying the laryngectomee to this session are also asked to provide feedback. If several instruments offer equally good results in terms of the acceptability of the speech produced, the decision should be made on the basis of sound quality, size of the instrument, ease of use, and personal preference. The decision should never be made on the basis of cost. Although pneumatic instruments have largely gone out of favor, primarily because of their bulk and the need to place one end over the stoma, they should not be ignored. The sound produced can be quite acceptable because it lacks the electronic sound of the others. Some patients use a pneumatic instrument with great skill. (The types of speech aids available were described in Chapter 4, and a listing of various models and their distributors is available in Appendix D.)

B. Instruction in the Use of Speech Aids

Instruction in the use of speech aids must be clear and uncomplicated. The clinician should be able to use the aids effectively to demonstrate their use. The exceptions to this are the pneumatic instrument, which requires the presence of a stoma, and the intraoral device, which must be made to the individual's oral specifications. Only by working with the instruments can the clinician get a clear understanding of the adjustments in placement of the unit, articulation, and rate of speech that are necessary to produce intelligible speech. Clinicians should be knowledgeable about the workings of the instrument so that simple troubleshooting can be done without returning the instrument to the manufacturer. This does not mean that clinicians should attempt to service malfunctioning parts. Manufacturer's instructions should be adhered to so as not to invalidate any warranties.

1. **Pneumatic devices** are infrequently used, primarily because of their bulkiness and the need to have access to the uncovered stoma. They also produce a very low pitch sound. Because the clinician is unable to demonstrate their use, the clinician must simply instruct the patient in what to do. The training film that accompanies the Tokyo artificial speech aid is also helpful.

a. **The cup end is placed firmly over the stom**a. It is important for a seal to be established so that air cannot leak around the cup. Stoma discs of the type used with the tracheoesophageal valve may be helpful. Demonstration of this placement takes place prior to asking the patient to attempt to produce sound. The patient is instructed to release the cup slightly from the stoma to inhale.

b. **With the cup end held firmly covering the stoma**, the patient is instructed to blow out a sound. (The mouthpiece is not used in this activity.) Progress to blowing two and then three sounds per breath, and stopping "voicing" between sounds.

c. The patient is then instructed to **attempt to change pitch by increasing air pressure**. This type of practice allows the patient to become adept at making sound and beginning to control that sound.

d. With the cup end over the stoma, instruct the patient to **place the mouthpiece into the mouth** and on top of the tongue.

e. After the patient understands the placement of the unit, **vowels should be attempted first, followed by words**.

2. **Neck-held instruments** come in a variety of models that differ in size, sound produced, and methods of pitch and volume control, but they all function on the principle of transmitting an electronically produced sound through the tissues of the neck and making it accessible to shaping by the articulators as shown in Figure 5–2. The following steps should be followed in teaching the use of one of these devices. (An educational videotape, available at no charge from Siemens, describes the use of the Servox instrument in addition to providing other information. See Appendix D.)

a. First, the **clinician demonstrates** the sound produced by the instrument without placement on the neck followed by a demonstration of how it sounds in speaking.

b. The **clinician palpates the patient's neck** to locate the most supple area and places the instrument there.

c. The **patient is instructed to count** as the clinician manipulates the button for sound production. It may be necessary to

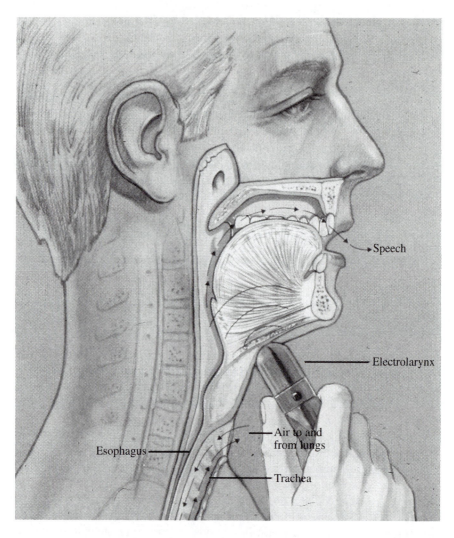

Speech

Electrolarynx

Air to and from lungs

Esophagus

Trachea

Figure 5–2. Representation of speech being produced with a neck-held instrument. (Photo courtesy of InHealth Corporation.)

try various areas on the neck to determine the site of best sound transmission. Typically, the best locations are under the jaw and just lateral to the midline of the neck. As placement moves closer to the ear on either side, less sound energy will be available in the vocal tract making the speech less intelligible. Sometimes it may be necessary to place the instrument on the cheek to get the clearest speech. The head of the instrument must be placed so that the full head is in contact with the skin. It is not necessary to press the instrument into the neck, but the seal must be complete between the skin and the head of the instrument to avoid the escape of sound around the edges of the instrument. When sound does escape, it is noisy and interferes with speech intelligibility.

d. The **patient is instructed to shape the words** as clearly as possible with his or her mouth but without overexaggerating articulatory movements.

e. The **patient is cautioned against forceful exhalation** accompanying the speech attempt. In using the instruments, the movement of the mouth to shape words is of primary importance, and this does not require any forceful expelling of air from the lungs. If the patient will be pursuing either prosthetically aided speech or esophageal speech, learning to extinguish the tendency to exhale forcefully to produce sound when using the instrument will prove helpful later.

f. If an acceptable sound is elicited, the **patient is then instructed in handling the instrument**. The use of a mirror can often be helpful as the patient attempts to identify the correct placement of the instrument. It is important not to flood the patient with all instructions at once. As the patient begins to experiment with the device, things will be discovered that may never need discussion or specific instruction. Information overload may confuse the patient. Many patients do well with instruments on their very first attempt following a short demonstration. Additional instruction can be given in increments as the patient experiments with this new form of speech. This instruction usually involves the following:

(1) recognition of the fact that **the finger and the mouth must be coordinated** so that speech and the sound begin and end simultaneously;

(2) learning to **turn off the sound during natural pauses** in speech, but not to make speech staccato by constant interruption of the sound for each word;

(3) learning to **reduce speech rate**; and

(4) learning to **increase the precision of articulation**.

g. When necessary, **instruction in articulation** should begin with the production of voiceless consonants. If the patient had a tendency to slight those sounds presurgically, they will probably be inaudible with the use of the electronic speech aids. Slight adjustments in the manner of articulation must be made for some of these sounds. For example, the laryngectomized individual cannot produce the sounds /s, f, θ, or ʃ/ with a continuous stream of air flow. The sounds must be produced by using the air within the mouth as short bursts of sound. Patients should be instructed to practice producing all voiceless consonants sharply.

h. Articulation practice may have to extend to **clear production of voiced sounds** as well. This is best done by having the patient practice words that contain a particular sound while using the instrument and listening carefully for that sound.

    (1) Instruction in phrasing may or may not be necessary. The clinician must continually assess the patient's skill in using the instrument. If a patient routinely keeps the sound on throughout long utterances, attention should be paid to interrupting the sound at the phrase break. If, on the other hand, a patient develops a staccato style of speech by interrupting the sound after every word, a flow of speech with continuous sound for entire phrases must be taught.

j. **Coordination between manual initiation and cessation of sound and the movement of the mouth** is vital. Speaking before starting the sound, continuing to speak after stopping the sound, starting the sound before the mouth starts to move, or keeping the sound on after completion of the utterance are behaviors that indicate poor coordination of speech and sound and will be detrimental to intelligibility of speech. When any of these behaviors is observed appropriate instruction must be given.

k. Attention should be paid to **nonverbal behaviors**. Patients should be encouraged to look directly at the person to whom they are speaking. Any extraneous or superfluous mannerisms should be eliminated quickly before they become established habits.

3. The **oral types of instruments** typically have a plastic tube which is placed in the mouth to introduce sound into the oral cavity where it is capable of being shaped into speech sounds. It may be necessary for patients to use this type of model if:

a. a slow healing **fistula** is present,

b. hard fibrous **scar tissue** is present and impedes transcutaneous sound transmission,

    c. the **buzz of the neck-held instrument** is too noisy because the noise source is close to the ear, or

    d. he or she has a preference for the sound of the instrument or the quality of the speech produced.

4. The following steps should be pursued in **teaching the use of the oral instrument**.

    a. The **clinician demonstrates** the sound the instrument produces with and without speech.

    b. The **clinician demonstrates placement of the oral tube**. Patients must be shown clearly that approximately 1 to 1½ inches of the tube must be placed within the mouth on top of the tongue. When the tube is not correctly placed, the clarity of speech will suffer. Patients will need to experiment with placement of the tube. It can be inserted from the corner of the mouth and lie across the tongue, or it can enter at the midpoint of the mouth. It is important that the tongue not block the tip of the tube.

    c. The patient experiments with the instrument. The clarity of articulation must be stressed, and the patient must not use forceful exhalation. The patient must learn to move his or her mouth as naturally as possible to produce clear speech. Patients often try to hold onto the tube with the tongue and the lips. This restricts the ability to move the articulators appropriately for sound placement and results in unintelligible speech.

    d. The same type of **practice on voiceless consonants** described above for neck-held instruments may be necessary for patients who choose an oral instrument. In addition, these patients must learn to produce sounds in the presence of a tube in the mouth. Some sounds (such as /s/) even require that the patient bite down on the tube.

    e. Factors of **coordination of the sound with the movement of the mouth**, cessation of sound for natural pauses, and reduced rate of speech must be discussed, demonstrated, and practiced.

    f. Nonverbal behaviors are important. Because the tube must be held in the mouth, it is easy for patients to hold their hand in front of the mouth as they speak. This should be guarded against because intelligibility of speech is reduced and the listener does not have the benefit of watching the speaker's mouth. Good eye contact should be maintained between the speaker and the listener.

5. Much of what has been discussed in teaching the use of the neck and mouth types of instruments pertains to the **intraoral device**. However, because the unit is contained in the mouth and has a remote control via a hand-held unit there are some unique features that will require attention. Among the most important are practicing control of the hand-held unit and coordination of sound activation with speech movements.

6. After the patient demonstrates a basic speaking proficiency with the speech aid, the clinician should instruct the patient in the **mechanics of the instrument**. The methods for making adjustments of volume and pitch, battery replacement and recharging, and routine maintenance of the device should be demonstrated so that the patient is able to use the speech aid with maximum independence.

IV. ESOPHAGEAL SPEECH

The previous chapter contained a description of the physiology of esophageal speech. The emphasis in this chapter is on teaching esophageal speech (see Figure 5–3).

A. Teaching Esophageal Speech

Teaching esophageal speech requires skill, understanding of the anatomy and physiology of esophageal sound production, patience, sensitivity to the psychological impact of the process on the patient, and the ability to be supportive. It is extremely helpful if the clinician has acquired the ability to produce esophageal sound. Often demonstration of its production can be more instructive than verbal explanations. When a clinician has not learned that skill, it may be helpful to provide team teaching with the assistance of a laryngectomized person who has acquired functional esophageal speech.

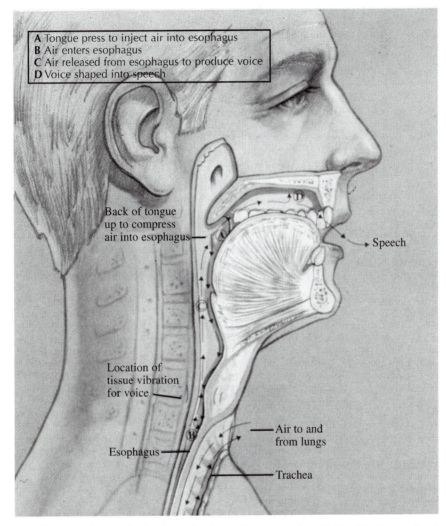

A Tongue press to inject air into esophagus
B Air enters esophagus
C Air released from esophagus to produce voice
D Voice shaped into speech

Back of tongue
up to compress
air into esophagus

Speech

Location of
tissue vibration
for voice

Air to and
from lungs

Esophagus

Trachea

Figure 5–3. Esophageal speech production. (Photo courtesy of InHealth Corporation.)

B. Learning Esophageal Speech

For the patient, learning esophageal speech requires a high degree of motivation, a willingness to learn to produce a sound voluntarily that has always had a negative stigma, patience, the physical integrity necessary to produce esophageal sound, emotional stability, and a host of other factors that are difficult to itemize.

C. Production of Esophageal Sound

Production of esophageal sound can be approached in various ways, and there are no set rules that can be applied to all patients. The basic tenet of our philosophy is to attempt to elicit production of esophageal sound in the simplest possible way. This rationale also guides the order of the methods. When a method is successful in eliciting a sound, we may continue to pursue that method or we may note this success but continue to explore the patient's response to other approaches. Patients are advised in advance that a variety of approaches will be tried. The goal is to find the method that works best for that individual and provides the best sound with the least effort.

D. Methods for Teaching Esophageal Sound Production and Speech

There are a variety of methods for teaching esophageal sound production and speech. Clinicians who are involved with this population of patients and this method of alaryngeal speech find that their style and favored methods of instruction evolve with experience. The following sections are based on clinical experience with methods that have proven effective as well as less successful methods.

1. The clinician should listen carefully for any **involuntary production of esophageal sound**. Some patients will inflate or charge the esophagus unconsciously as they attempt to produce whispered speech. Others may spontaneously use the inhalation method (see Chapter 4) and produce occasional sound nonvolitionally and with little conscious awareness of what they have done. Even if the clinician does not hear evidence of such sounds during the first session, patients should be asked if they have made any sounds involuntarily since their surgery and, if they have, to describe when it happened. It is sometimes possible to capitalize on such instances of involuntary sound production by asking the patient to "do it again."

2. Ask the patient to **make a burping sound**. It is always good for the clinician to be able to demonstrate production of a "burp." This may make the patient more comfortable about producing a sound that has been considered socially unacceptable. Some patients will be able to produce such a sound with ease. The clinician should carefully observe the manner in which the patient attempts to produce the burp, whether successful or not. It is especially important to note whether the patient is working hard

at swallowing during the attempt. If that is the case, it is a behavior that should not be encouraged or reinforced. If the patient seems to be injecting air into the esophagus appropriately and producing sound, the clinician should continue with additional trials during which the patient's attention is directed at determining how the sound is being produced.

3. The clinician should **demonstrate injection of air** in an audible manner and ask the patient to produce a similar sound. The sound is typically referred to as a "klunk," and should be audible but not excessively loud. Some patients who may not have understood or known instinctively how to produce a voluntary burp may be able to imitate this maneuver. If they can, they are instructed to try to reverse that action as soon as the air is injected by opening the mouth immediately to say /a/. Once again, demonstration is more instructive than verbal description.

4. Try to **trigger esophageal sound production using plosive consonants**. The patient is instructed to say /ta ta ta/ repetitively. The clinician should do this along with the patient and demonstrate the production of a hard /t/ sound by pressing the tongue against the alveolar ridge. The clinician should gradually introduce easy air injection and production of esophageal sound into the string of repetitions of /ta/ and provide a model for the patient. Patients may sometimes charge the esophagus sufficiently while producing the string of /ta/s to produce an esophageal sound. Others may begin to inject air into the esophagus actively and produce esophageal sound. If either of these occur, the clinician should reinforce the behavior by having the patient repeat it. The same activity can be tried with repetitions of /pa/ and /ka/. A word of caution about the use of /ka/. If the patient produces a sound triggered by repetition of /ka/ the clinician must listen carefully to be sure that it is not a pharyngeally produced sound rather than an esophageally produced sound. The perceptual characteristics of these two sounds differ. The pharyngeal sound is produced higher in the hypopharynx and has the "Donald Duck" sound. If the patient is producing sound in this manner, it would be best to avoid the use of the /ka/ as a trigger. Production of pharyngeal sound should be strongly discouraged. It is very difficult to change when it becomes habitual and it leads to very poor speech production.

5. **Explain how esophageal sound is produced**. It is often helpful for patients to have an understanding of what they are trying to

do, or what they are doing, in the production of esophageal sound. It is best, however, not to introduce this intellectual and conceptual analysis too early in the process. Simple diagrammatic pictures of the anatomy and physiology for sound production before and after surgery (see Figure 4–6), or the use of three-dimensional models, can be helpful. A simplified verbal explanation of how the anatomy is changed and what those changes mean for the way sound is produced helps patients understand why the esophagus must be charged with air and why the activity for speaking no longer involves pushing air from the lungs.

6. The patient can learn to **manipulate the air trapped in the mouth** by puffing his or her cheeks out and by moving the air around in the mouth from side to side and forward. The patient is then instructed to let that air move quickly back to enter the esophagus easily. If the patient can do this successfully, he or she is encouraged to do it repetitively a few times before the idea of bringing that air back up as sound is introduced.

7. In addition to using the voiceless stop plosive/vowel combinations noted above to trigger esophageal sound production, there are a number of **words that often trigger sound production**. Among the most commonly used are: *scotch, church, skate, stop,* and *scratch.* It is important for the clinician to note whether esophageal sound is triggered on the vowels in those words in addition to the audible production of the voiceless consonants. In trying this approach patients should be instructed to say the words repetitively. The intent is to trigger insufflation of the esophagus.

8. As a last resort, after having tried and retried all of the above methods to teach injection, the "idea" of **swallowing** in a controlled way may be introduced. The patient is instructed to take a very small sip of water, hold it in the mouth momentarily, and then swallow it, being conscious of where the water seems to enter the esophagus. In this way the patient is helped to feel where the injected air is supposed to go. This act may be repeated several times. The patient may then be instructed to try to produce a sound immediately after swallowing the water. The progression for patients in using this technique must be to wean them away from the swallowing of the water as quickly as possible, and attempt to change that action to an injection rather than a swallow. Another technique using the swallow method is

to have the patient swallow a sip of water and immediately produce a very quick second swallow followed by an attempt to produce sound. This second swallow may be more like an injection than a true swallow. It must be done quickly and immediately after the first swallow. If the patient is using injection, that behavior should be reinforced by having the patient attend to the difference between the two "swallows" and then learn to do only the second type.

9. The **inhalation method** is described by many authors and is used by some esophageal speakers interchangeably with the injection method. The usual instructions and descriptions given to the patient when teaching the inhalation method include sniffing air in or pulling air into the mouth, nose, and throat. Patients can be instructed to yawn as naturally as possible, a behavior that often triggers nonvolitional opening of the pharyngoesophageal (PE) segment allowing air to enter the esophagus. This can often be detected as a click at the most open part of the yawn. If this occurs, the patient is then instructed to attempt to produce sound as the air is pushed out of the esophagus.

10. A **three-step maneuver** is also used to teach the inhalation method. The patient is instructed to exhale through the stoma, to cover the stoma with a finger, and with the stoma covered to suck air quickly into the mouth and throat. Often a sound will be produced as air is "inhaled" in this manner. When this is noted, the patient should be instructed to do the maneuver with less force and to attempt to reverse the direction of the air immediately so that a sound can be made on "exhalation."

We have had little success in teaching the inhalation method despite many years of experience teaching alaryngeal speech. Patients often have difficulty conceptualizing what they are asked to do. The very term "inhalation" and the words used to describe how the sound is made seem to increase the tendency for stoma blasting. Even when patients are successful in producing the sound, they often have difficulty in forming the sound into words. There have been a number of patients who have spontaneously, nonvolitionally, and without the benefit of therapy adopted the inhalation method. Unfortunately, the sound was inconsistent and produced with no awareness of how it was being done. They experienced great difficulty in developing that awareness and learning volitional control over its production. Indeed, in most of these cases it was necessary to extinguish this behavior and replace it with injection, which they were able to control.

11. **Extending sound production into speech** early in the process is helpful to patients, but it should not be rushed. It is essential to build a solid foundation for production of functional esophageal speech. That foundation is based on the ability to produce sound consistently, with ease, and with minimal latency between charging the esophagus and producing sound. Patients should be able to produce /uh/, /ah/, /pa, ka, sa, cha, wa, fa/ or any other CV unit with equal ease, repetitively, rapidly, and consistently. When the patient is able to do this, production of words and sentences should follow with relative ease.

   a. Some patients encounter no difficulty in producing syllables or words that begin with a **consonant that occludes the oral cavity** such as /p, t, k, tʃ, ʃ/ and so forth, but they encounter difficulty with vowels, or less closed consonants such as /w, y, r/. When that is the case, the patient must be reminded of the need to charge the esophagus prior to attempting production of the speech unit.

   b. Begin with the practice of single syllable words and have the patient produce a given word repeatedly just as he or she did with the consonant/vowel segments. As the patient progresses through many words, note whether there is a pattern to words that present difficulty, particularly whether the initial consonant is a factor.

   c. As the patient progresses to longer units of speech, it is important that sound is present on each syllable of each word. Patients must learn to sense how far they can go on the available air supply. Although it is sometimes necessary to instruct a patient to try to say more than a single syllable on one injection of air, it is often the case that patients begin to do this quite automatically as they become adept at controlling injection and sound production. However, the opposite is more likely, and the patient attempts to say more than he or she is capable of with a limited air supply.

   d. Slowing the rate of speech and becoming used to the slower rate is one of the most difficult things for a laryngectomee to learn. Rather than focusing on rate, focusing on the clarity of each word and on appropriate phrasing will result in a slowing of the overall speaking rate.

E. Problem Areas

There are a number of problems that interfere with the acquisition of functional esophageal speech or detract from its acceptability. Some may be temporary, some require further assessment, and some require changing habits.

1. Patients undergoing **radiation therapy** may have difficulty producing esophageal speech and experience a slower rate of progress. This is usually temporary and reflects the various effects of radiation therapy. Some of the problems may be caused by dryness in the throat and mouth, fatigue, pain, swelling, and very thick mucus. Some patients must temporarily discontinue therapy because of the severity of these effects. The speech-language pathologist must recognize these problems, have patience, adjust the short-term goals appropriately, and explain their effects to the patient to prevent discouragement.

2. **The patient who cannot produce esophageal sound** despite the apparent ability to inject air presents a challenge. Any of the following factors may be involved.

   a. **Excessive tension** during attempted production of esophageal sound may be evidenced by a lack of mouth opening and the tongue held high in the back of the mouth, holding the breath or excessive force of pulmonary exhalation, clenching the fists, and other observable signs of tension. Psychologically, the patient may be reluctant to produce this type of sound.

   b. **Lack of any muscle activity to expel air**. The patient injects and simply opens the mouth.

   c. **Hypotonic PE segment**. The patient may lack adequate tonicity in the PE segment or the vocal tract resulting in very weak sound production. It may be helpful to explore whether the sound can be improved if the patient applies digital pressure to the neck during sound production. It is necessary for the patient to apply this fairly gentle pressure in different locations, usually superior and slightly lateral to the stoma, and locate the ideal spot. If this digital pressure is helpful it is almost immediately apparent by the production of a much louder and improved sound. Patients will need to practice using this pressure to learn how to place the finger in the appropriate spot quickly and apply the needed amount of pressure.

d. **Spasm or hypertonicity of the PE segment.** The speech-language pathologist can perform an insufflation test (see Chapter 6) to determine if there is hypertonicity of the PE segment. The absence of relatively fluent sound production during insufflation suggests a diminished capability for vibratory activity of the PE segment. Most often this is due to hypertonicity or spasm of the PE segment. Other causes include stricture, stenosis, post-radiation edema, or tumor recurrence. If insufflation is failed, the patient should be referred to the surgeon for consideration of a videoradiographic study and/or lidocaine injection that results in a pharyngeal plexus nerve block to confirm the presence of PE spasm or hypertonicity before recommending a pharyngeal relaxation procedure. The speech-language pathologist should be present during the radiographic study. Videofluoroscopy should be used to examine the patient at rest, while swallowing, during attempts at injection of air, and during insufflation testing. These tasks should be repeated during lidocaine block of the pharyngeal plexus. Improvement in voicing during nerve block suggests hypertonicity or spasm of the PE segment. Pharyngeal constrictor relaxation procedures, including pharyngeal constrictor myotomy, neurectomy, or semi-permanent chemical denervation through the use of botulinum toxin injections, are generally successful in the management of hypertonicity or spasm to achieve acceptable vocal productions.

e. **The patient who cannot inject** or charge the esophagus in any manner should be evaluated for possible spasm of the PE segment in much the same manner as described for assessment of the hypertonic PE segment in the preceding section.

f. **A loud klunk** is often indicative of rapid and tense injection of air. It can be disruptive to the listener when it is so obvious as to detract from the patient's speech.

g. **Multiple injections** disrupt the flow of speech, make the person appear to be gasping for air, and are unnecessary for the production of sound. It is very easy for patients to develop the habit of multiple injections. In their early attempts at producing sound, they may not be successful on the first injection and must try again. It is a habit that should be marked for elimination as soon as it is observed. Because there is no esophageal reservoir for air to be stored, most of the injected air in multiple charges simply goes down to the stomach and is of no use for speech.

h. **Excessive stoma blast** occurs as a result of attempting to use pulmonary air for speech. It is highly distracting, a sign of excessive effort and strain, and detracts from the quality of the esophageal sound produced. It is a difficult behavior to change, but it must be changed early in the process. The patient can be made aware of stoma blast in a number of ways, for example, holding a hand in front of the stoma to feel the air, using a microphone or other system to amplify the sound of the blast, becoming aware of the sensations of pushing that accompany it, and so forth. Although esophageal speech is coordinated with the expiratory cycle, this is a natural—not forced—exhalation, that parallels the production of sound in the esophagus.

i. **Intrusive consonant sounds** may occur when a patient has learned to inject using a consonant. For example, a person may seem to be able to inject only on /ta/ and will start every word with a /t/ sound whether or not it should be there. This may be true also of the person who has learned to inject with the lips closed and can only do so in this manner. Thus, the listener anticipates hearing a word that begins with a bilabial consonant. This pattern is very distracting to the listener. In earlier sections we stressed the need for patients to learn to inject in various ways, regardless of the initial consonant sound.

j. **Grimaces and extraneous head movements** should be avoided. Head bobbing is often seen when patients are beginning to produce esophageal speech. Any facial or head movements that are not a part of speech production should be eliminated. The use of a mirror during practice can be helpful. Patients should maintain good eye contact with the person being addressed.

k. **Talking on the telephone** is often a stumbling block for the laryngectomee. Too often, initial attempts may be met with the sound of a click because the unwitting person at the other end hangs up. It is wise for laryngectomees to arrange their first use of the telephone with a family member or friend as a practice session or trial run. It is important for them to learn techniques that prevent people hanging up. One suggestion is to make an immediate request that the person not hang up and then explain the different sound of the voice. All laryngectomees, regardless of their type of alaryngeal speech, do best with the phone mouthpiece positioned toward the nose. This eliminates stoma noise, the buzz of an electrolarynx, or the sound of the tracheostoma valve closing.

CHAPTER

6

Tracheoesophageal Speech

I. INTRODUCTION

Tracheoesophageal speech is not just a method of speech. The speech is the end result of a process that begins with a surgical procedure (described in Chapter 4). Next it involves the fitting of a prosthesis, instruction in its use and care, instruction in speech production, and skilled problem solving. The process is typically handled by a team comprising a surgeon and a speech-language pathologist. Special training and skills are required in order to provide appropriate services to the patient and to protect both the patient and the speech-language pathologist from harm. (Guidelines for Evaluation and Treatment for Tracheoesophageal Fistulization/Puncture, *Asha, 36* [Suppl. 7], 1992.)

As discussed in Chapter 4, tracheoesophageal puncture (TEP) can be performed as a primary procedure at the time of laryngectomy, or as a delayed or secondary procedure. It is a viable method of voice restoration with relatively few limitations. All speech-language pathologists involved in the selection of patients and the fitting of voice prostheses should adhere strictly to the Universal Precautions to prevent the risk of disease transmission from blood-borne pathogens. These are contained in the *Centers for Disease Control Morbidity and Mortality Weekly Report* (Centers for Disease Control, 1988) or ASHA's *AIDS/HIV Update* (American Speech-Language-Hearing Association, 1990). Prosthesis fitting should be performed only in a medical setting where adequate support services are available.

II. PATIENT SELECTION

Patient selection for primary TEP is usually determined by the surgeon, whose main concern is with tumor control and a minimum of complications. TEP is typically delayed if extended reconstruction of the pharynx or esophagus is required, if the patient's general health is compromised, or an extended recovery period is anticipated. The speech-language pathologist should be involved in selecting patients for primary TEP by providing input about the patient's motivation, manual dexterity, adequacy of eyesight, emotional stability, general hygiene habits, and alertness. The candidacy factors discussed below should be employed by the team in selecting patients for secondary puncture.

A. Candidacy Factors

1. **Healing from previous surgery** should be complete—typically a minimum of 6 weeks after surgery.

2. **Radiation therapy** or other forms of treatment should be completed, including a sufficient period of recovery from the effects of such treatments (usually 6 weeks).

3. The patient should have **an adequate interval of being free of disease.**

4. The patient should be **medically stable** in areas other than the laryngectomy. Patients must have adequate air volume and adequate ability to generate the air pressures required to move air through the prosthesis and generate sound. The introduction of low resistance prostheses has enabled many laryngectomees with respiratory problems to become successful TEP speakers.

5. The **tracheostoma must be of adequate size** (1.5 cm minimum) to house the prosthesis, and it must be above the jugular notch at the manubrium. If the stoma has a tendency to stenose, the patient may need to wear a silicone laryngectomy (tracheostoma) tube (Figure 6–1) that is windowed to accommodate the prosthesis, be fitted with a prosthesis that is built into a laryngectomy tube (Bivona-Colorado™) (Figure 6–1), or undergo surgical stoma revision (stomaplasty). An excessively large stoma may be difficult to occlude manually.

6. There must be a **healthy common wall** between the trachea and esophagus to accommodate the prosthesis.

7. The patient should display **emotional stability** sufficient to undergo the surgical procedure followed by fitting of a device and training in its use. Dependence on drugs or alcohol to the extent that the patient is unable to keep scheduled appointments or adequately maintain the device would eliminate the patient from consideration.

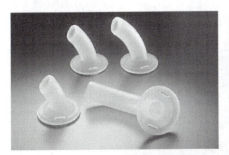
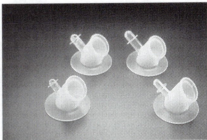
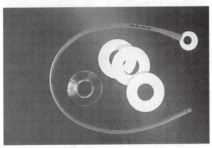

Figure 6–1. Upper left panel: Tracheostoma vent (Photo courtesy of Bivona), **Upper right panel:** Colorado Voice Prosthesis (Photo courtesy of Bivona), **Lower center panel:** Blom-Singer insufflation test kit. (Photo courtesy of InHealth Corporation.)

8. The patient should display a **degree of motivation** sufficient to follow through with the complete program of voice restoration, distinct from his or her family members' desire to see the patient achieve improved communication.

9. The patient's **eyesight, manual dexterity and control, habits of general hygiene, and general alertness** must be considered. If the patient has problems in any of these areas, it is necessary to determine whether a spouse or other caregiver is available and capable of assuming these responsibilities. The introduction of extended wear prostheses has enabled a greater number of laryngectomees to pursue the option of tracheoesophageal speech, because the requirements for routine care of these devices are minimal.

10. The prospective candidate for TEP, having met the above qualifications, should then undergo **insufflation testing**. This procedure is within the scope of practice of the speech-language pathologist who has the appropriate competencies. The procedure involves the transnasal insertion of a rubber catheter past the pharyngoesophageal junction, introduction of air into the esophagus through the catheter, and production of sound. A judgment of the adequacy and quality of the sound that is elicited must be made.

   a. **The Blom-Singer® insufflation test kit** (see Figure 6–1) contains a measured section of 14 French red rubber catheter attached to a tracheostoma adapter and housing. To perform the test, the housing is affixed to the stomal area of the neck. After coating the catheter tip with a water-soluble lubricant, it is passed transnasally so that the marker at the 25 cm point rests at the nasal tip. It is sometimes helpful to ask the patient to swallow as the catheter is slowly advanced to prevent coiling of the catheter in the pharynx. If the catheter is not inserted fully beyond the PE segment, the test may be invalid. The catheter is secured to the nose with adhesive tape and the tracheostoma adapter is attached to the housing. The patient is instructed to inhale, and with the clinician manually covering the tracheostoma adapter, he or she is asked to open his or her mouth as if to say /a/ and begin to slowly exhale, thus self-insufflating the esophagus. The patient should be able to produce sound easily. A high-pitched, strained vocal quality or reduced fluency of production is regarded as insufflation failure. Ideally, production of a vowel should be sustained for a minimum of 8 seconds, and the patient should be able to count to 15 on a single breath. These trials should be without excessive strain or tension, and free of attempts to pump in or swallow air that would prevent release of the pulmonary air. When the initial test is unsuccessful, repeated trials may be attempted. A slight repositioning of the catheter will sometimes meet with success. Some laryngectomees present with extreme anxiety concerning their potential for oral communication and will fail insufflation testing in the presence of a viable PE segment until the emotional reaction associated with the testing procedure can be overcome. Care should be taken to avoid numerous unsuccessful trials, because the patient will begin to complain of abdominal distention and excess gas.

b. **Unsuccessful insufflation testing** should lead to referral for further explanation of the causes for failure. Some possible causes include stricture, fibrosis, radiation edema, tumor recurrence, or PE spasm or hypertonicity. Therefore, the decision to undergo a pharyngeal constrictor relaxation procedure should not be made on the basis of a failed insufflation test alone. A videoradiographic study (see Figure 6–2) and/ or lidocaine injection for pharyngeal plexus nerve block to induce relaxation of the PE segment are helpful in making the differential diagnosis. The videofluoroscopic study should be performed in the presence of the speech-language pathologist and should include examination of the structures at rest, during swallow, and during insufflation testing. These tasks are repeated following lidocaine injection. Successful insufflation under the nerve block condition suggests hypertonicity or spasm. This can usually be managed by one of the PE relaxation procedures: pharyngeal constrictor myotomy, pharyngeal plexus neurectomy, or periodic chemical denervation through the use of botulinum toxin injections. These are generally successful in the management of hypertonicity or spasm to achieve fluent vocal productions.

11. **Preoperative recording of intraesophageal peak pressure levels** has been proposed by Lewin, Baugh, and Baker (1987) as a procedure that can more objectively assess the response of the PE segment to air insufflation and aid in predicting success of TEP. It is reported to be more than 90% accurate. Patients

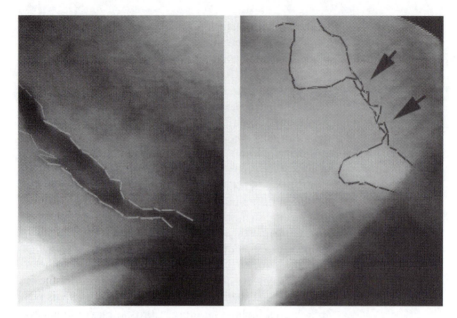

Figure 6–2. Left: Videoradiographic study showing absence of pharyngeal constrictor spasm on swallow. **Right:** Same patient showing pharyngeal constrictor spasm on attempting to phonate.

found to have intermediate or high intraesophageal pressures required pharyngeal constrictor relaxation to become fluent tracheoesophageal speakers.

B. Timing Considerations

Timing for fitting the voice prosthesis may be different for each patient. Clearance from the otolaryngologist should be obtained before proceeding with the fitting procedure to ensure proper healing of the puncture site and surrounding tissues.

1. For the patient with a **primary TEP** (puncture performed at the time of laryngectomy), fitting the prosthesis may be delayed for 10 days to 3 weeks or until surgical sites show adequate healing. The stenting catheter should slide easily in the puncture tract. If there is considerable resistance to movement of the catheter, wait an additional day or more before fitting the prosthesis. The presence of a draining fistula, indicative of incomplete healing of the suture lines, is a con-

traindication for fitting the voice prosthesis. In the case of a primary puncture, the catheter used to stent the surgically created puncture may double as a feeding tube. In this case, the patient should be eating well by mouth before fitting the prosthesis, or placement of a nasogastric feeding tube will be necessary to maintain nutrition.

2. Fitting the prosthesis for the patient with **secondary TEP** (a separate surgical procedure any time after laryngectomy) may take place anywhere from 48 hours to 1 week or more after the procedure. A slightly longer time is allowed for patients who have undergone a pharyngeal constrictor myotomy. The puncture must be healed well without tenderness or erythema of the puncture site prior to the fitting. The stenting catheter should slide easily in the puncture tract. If there is considerable resistance to movement of the catheter, wait an additional day or more before fitting the prosthesis. Occasionally when a pharyngeal constrictor myotomy is performed as part of the puncture procedure, a fistula of the neck will develop, indicating incomplete healing of the operative site in the neck. Prosthesis fitting should be delayed in these cases until the fistula has completely healed as confirmed by videofluoroscopy. In the interim, the patient should be restricted to nonoral nutrition, and the puncture catheter is used as a feeding tube.

3. In some cases, an **extended wear prosthesis** may be inserted in the puncture site intraoperatively as part of the TEP procedure. The surgeon will determine the proper length of the prosthesis by measuring the depth of the tracheoesophageal wall with a slight allowance made for potential postoperative edema. The speech-language pathologist is responsible for teaching the patient the method of achieving voice and the maintenance of the device. Typically the patient is asked to limit the amount of talking for the first 1–2 days until sufficient healing has occurred.

III. FITTING THE PROSTHESIS

A. Procedure

The procedure for fitting is usually consistent from one patient to another. An overview of the entire procedure should be provided and the patient should be informed about what is about to be done prior to each step in the process.

1. To **remove the catheter**, it may be necessary to remove the sutures that were placed at the time of surgery. This may be performed by the otolaryngologist, nurse, or speech-language pathologist (assuming that there has been adequate training in this procedure). If a urethral catheter has been used as a feeding tube, the balloon may be inflated at its distal tip. In this case, the residual air should be withdrawn from the catheter balloon using a 10-cc syringe prior to removing the catheter. The stenting catheter is removed part way while the area is thoroughly cleaned. Mucus crusts should be removed with a forceps (tweezers) after they are loosened by the application of a surgical sponge coated with hydrogen peroxide. Care should be taken to avoid dripping into the airway. A clean 16 French catheter, knotted or plugged at the proximal end to prevent regurgitation of esophageal contents and lightly coated with a water-soluble surgical lubricant, replaces the stenting catheter and is held in place by tape. As the catheter is inserted, the angle of the puncture tract is observed. Whenever a catheter or prosthesis is not in place, the patient is cautioned not to swallow to avoid aspiration of saliva through the puncture tract. The puncture should not remain unstented without a catheter or prosthesis for more than a few seconds at a time.

2. To **dilate the puncture tract**, the 16 French catheter is left in place for a brief period of time (usually about 10 minutes) until it slides easily in the puncture tract. At this time it is replaced with a new 18 French catheter which has been prepared for insertion. Typically a 16 French prosthesis will be used initially after surgery. Dilation to 18 French will allow for ease of insertion of the 16 French prosthesis. If the decision has been made on a subsequent visit to use a prosthesis of 20 French diameter, the puncture should be dilated to 22 French to allow ease of insertion. Dilation should proceed in a step-by-step fashion, increasing the catheter size incrementally only after the catheter currently stenting the puncture slides easily in the tract to avoid unnecessary tissue trauma, separation of the tracheoesophageal common wall with entrance into the anterior mediastinum, or incomplete insertion of the prosthesis through the puncture. In some cases, dilation to the appropriate diameter may require stenting

overnight. In this case, make certain that the catheter is inserted approximately half its length and is firmly secured with tape to the neck. Punctures that are slow to dilate are in no way indicative of future failure with tracheoesophageal speech and usually are reflective of healthy tissue of the tracheoesophageal wall.

3. To **test the phonatory mechanism** with the least possible resistance to airflow, check voicing with an **open tract** (without the stenting catheter or prosthesis in the puncture tract). To do this, the catheter is slowly removed and the patient is reminded not to swallow. The patient inhales a moderate amount, then as the clinician occludes the stoma, the patient is asked to phonate /a/. This should result in sound production. After a few trials, the catheter is replaced and the fitting can proceed.

   a. If **no sound is produced** after several trials, the catheter should be replaced or a dummy prosthesis inserted, and the fitting should be postponed for a few days to allow for additional time for healing and reduction of edema.

   b. For **patients who have been speaking well with the prosthesis** and who subsequently develop voice difficulty, the open tract test is helpful to distinguish between problems of the vibrating segment versus the prosthesis. Typically the best voice that the patient will hope to achieve is the open tract voice, because airflow is unobstructed by the prosthesis. A further discussion of the possible causes of post-fitting aphonia and suggested solutions can be found in Section IX, Problem Solving.

4. To **determine correct prosthesis length**, a **sizing device**, available from the manufacturer, is used. When the dilating catheter slides easily in the puncture tract, it is removed and the measuring probe, coated with a light film of surgical lubricant, is inserted. It is possible to sense the retention collar unfold as it passes completely through the tract and into the esophagus. It is also possible to feel when the probe can go no further as it impinges on the posterior esophageal wall. At that point, the clinician should gently retract the measuring device slightly away from the posterior wall pointing it downward toward the esophagus. It is then retracted further until the flange is just behind the anterior esophageal wall and resistance to further retraction is felt. The sizing instru-

ment should gently rotate 360° in the tract. If resistance is felt, the device may not be fully inserted through the tract. The procedure up to this point, beginning with dilation, should be repeated.

5. When the sizing device is comfortably within the esophageal lumen, neither abutting against the posterior wall nor too snugly pulled against the anterior esophageal wall, the **measurement is taken**.

   a. It is better to **measure too long rather than too short**, otherwise the prosthesis will not be fully inserted into the esophagus. This can result in closure of the puncture from the esophageal side.

   b. It is sometimes helpful to leave the sizing device in place for a minute or two while the **patient swallows**. On occasion, the probe will be pushed forward slightly by the swallow. It may be more comfortable for the patient to fit the prosthesis allowing for this adjustment as long as the prosthesis is in the esophagus and is sufficiently long to maintain an open tract.

   c. The **measuring device is removed** and the dilating catheter is replaced.

6. The properly sized **prosthesis is selected**. The 16 French duckbill prosthesis is often used for the initial fitting. The smaller diameter is preferable until the puncture site matures. The contour of the distal tip of the duckbill type makes for smooth insertion in the freshly punctured mucosal tract. Additionally, the distal tip of the duckbill device offers a slightly longer extension of the prosthesis into the esophagus. This will help guard against underfitting and stenosis of the esophageal end of the puncture should post-fitting edema occur. However, due to its higher resistance to airflow, this prosthesis may not offer optimum voicing for many patients.

   a. **After additional healing** of the puncture has occurred, the clinician may select a different prosthesis style that will maximize the aerodynamic characteristics for tracheoesophageal voice production, ease of insertion and durability.

7. In **preparation for prosthesis insertion**, the valving mechanism is inspected for ease of opening and closing by squeezing gently on the prosthesis shaft.

a. The **prosthesis is placed on its inserter** and prepared with a light film of surgical lubricant.

b. The dilating catheter is checked once again for its ease of movement in the tract and removed, after reminding the patient not to swallow. If the patient will eventually be **independently changing the prosthesis** on a regular basis, he or she is asked to observe the clinician carefully performing these procedures, as well as to attend to the sensation when the retention collar flange clears the tracheoesophageal wall and unfolds into the esophagus.

c. The **prosthesis is inserted into the puncture** following the angle of the tract until the opening of the esophageal retention collar is felt (sometimes described as a "pop") and then retracted slightly so that the outer flange is flush against the posterior tracheal wall. The anterior end of the prosthesis should lie fairly flush against the puncture aperture.

d. While still attached to the insertion tool, the prosthesis is gently rotated 360° in the tract to confirm its proper placement. If **resistance is felt** or the prosthesis strap curls up on the inserter, the device may not be completely through the tract and insertion should be repeated, with additional dilation time, if necessary.

e. **When correct placement has been achieved**, the strap is grasped and released from the insertion tool. Holding on to the strap with one hand, the tool itself is then gently rotated and simultaneously withdrawn from the prosthesis with the other hand. To avoid possible aspiration of the prosthesis, it is important to hold on to the strap until the prosthesis is in place and the insertion tool is withdrawn. It should then be directed upward and taped to the neck above the stoma.

8. With the prosthesis in place, **check for any signs of leakage** around the puncture by having the patient swallow small amounts of water or other liquid. Observing the swallow with a light directed into the stoma will make it possible to detect leakage.

a. If **leakage around the prosthesis** is noted, wait approximately 20 minutes to see if the dilated puncture will close down around the prosthesis. Repeat the swallow testing and if leakage continues it suggests that the elasticity of the tracheoesophageal wall tissue may be compromised (particularly in cases where the peristomal area has been heavily radiated). The prosthesis should be removed and replaced with a 14 French catheter for several days until the puncture closes down around it.

b. If **leakage through the prosthesis** is observed, it should be checked for malfunction or incorrect placement.

c. Prostheses with hinged valves should first be evaluated in place by directing a bright **light through the prosthesis lumen** to inspect for adequate closure of the valving mechanism. If the hinged valve appears to be **stuck in the open position**, repeated dry swallows will usually correct the problem.

d. In any case, if **leakage persists**, the prosthesis should be removed, inspected closely for manufacturing defects, and replaced.

For more extensive explanation of leakage and other problems see Section IX on Problem Solving later in this chapter.

B. Fitting the Extended Wear Prostheses

The various **extended wear prostheses** are typically made of stiffer silicone or other materials and incorporate larger flanges to improve the retention capabilities of the device for long term placement. This necessitates a modification of the insertion process so as to reduce trauma to the tracheoesophageal tissues. The reader should consult with the manufacturer regarding the proper insertion techniques for any device.

1. The original Provox® prosthesis (Figure 4–9) and the Groningen device are **placed in a retrograde fashion**. In this technique, a special insertion tool (or catheter) is inserted into the puncture tract at the stoma and advanced upward to exit the mouth. The prosthesis is then affixed to the insertion device at the mouth. By gently retracting the insertion tool at the stoma, the prosthesis is drawn through the oropharynx and into the puncture tract. This procedure can be uncomfortable for many patients, necessitating the use of topical anesthesia to reduce gagging. This placement technique is useful, however, when there is a separation of the tracheoesophageal party wall and concern that the prosthesis may not go completely through the puncture tract using the standard "front-loading"

insertion technique. Removal of these devices is accomplished by pushing the prosthesis out the mouth with the insertion tool.

2. The InHealth® Indwelling device (Figure 4–10) utilizes a **gelatin capsule insertion** system. In this technique, the esophageal retention collar is folded into half of a gelatin capsule using a special loading tool. This results in a contoured tip, similar to the distal end of the duckbill prosthesis, to enable a smooth insertion into the tracheoesophageal passage. Within minutes after placement, the gelatin capsule dissolves in response to swallowed saliva or liquid, and the retention collar opens into the esophageal lumen. The usual "pop" that is felt as the retention collar passes through the puncture and opens into the esophagus with insertion of the duckbill or standard low resistance devices is absent with Gel Cap insertion. Extra care should be taken to ensure that the device is correctly placed. Confirmation of correct placement may be obtained with nasendoscopic visualization (See Appendix A) or fluoroscopy. Removal is accomplished by grasping the device with a locking hemostat and pulling it forward from the TE puncture tract.

3. The Provox2® prosthesis (Figure 4–9) is inserted by folding the prosthesis in a special **tapered insertion tube** and pushing it into the puncture tract with a plunger in a "front-loading" fashion. The puncture must be adequately dilated to accommodate opening of the insertion tube for release of the prosthesis into the tract and the inserter should be well lubricated. The use of a topical anesthetic is helpful to reduce patient discomfort. The prosthesis is removed by pushing it into the esophagus and allowing it to pass through the digestive tract, or it can be dislodged through the stoma with the use of a locking forceps.

IV. TRACHEOESOPHAGEAL VOICE PRODUCTION

A. Procedure

When correct placement and proper functioning of the prosthesis has been verified, the patient is instructed in the **method of voice production**.

1. Initially, the patient is instructed to inhale a moderate amount and attempt to **phonate while the clinician manually oc-**

cludes the stoma. The first few trials should consist of easy productions, such as vowel prolongations or counting. On these initial attempts, it is not unusual for the patient to inhale too deeply, thereby overinflating the esophagus, or to not activate the airflow correctly due to excess tension. Either of these will inhibit the production of sound.

2. If the patient has **previously learned esophageal speech** and attempts to begin each tracheoesophageal production with an air charge, voicing will not occur. The patient should be instructed to begin each voicing attempt with a widely open mouth until the air charging habit can be extinguished.

3. Some patients (and/or their caregivers) experience a dramatic **emotional response**, either positively or negatively, to these initial attempts to achieve voice. Laryngectomees who have had a prolonged recovery period and have been without functional oral communication for a considerable amount of time may be overwhelmed at the sudden ability to speak again. Others may feel that it is "not like their old voice" and express frustration with the perceived differences. If this occurs, it is important for the clinician to remind the patient that these initial attempts may not be representative of the eventual vocal quality that will be attained with practice and refinement of the tracheoesophageal voice. In either case, the clinician should allow ample time for the patient to express these emotions before proceeding with further vocal attempts.

4. The patient should then be taught to use a thumb or finger to **occlude the stoma manually**.

   a. A trial-and-error process may be required to discover which finger works best and the proper placement angle to **prevent air escape from the stoma**. A mirror can be helpful in training correct and consistent placement. It is important that the stoma be completely occluded, but the pressure against it should remain gentle. Usually, the tracheostoma can be observed to move slightly forward to meet the finger as speech is attempted.

   b. **Excessive inward pressure** may occlude the lumen of the prosthesis and prevent air from flowing through it.

   c. Excessive digital **pressure superior to the stoma rim** may result in kinking of the esophagus and impede the free flow of air that is necessary for vibration of the esophageal tissue. A slight downward pressure is usually best.

   d. Initial attempts at digital occlusion of the stoma are usually made with direct contact of the **finger against the stoma** until the laryngectomee consistently attains the correct placement "by feel."

   e. After this training stage, the patient should be encouraged to perform stoma **occlusion over a stoma cover**. This will be less cumbersome and distracting, and more hygienic. It may require experimentation with various fabrics to achieve optimum closure.

   f. For **irregularly shaped or large stomas**, creative ingenuity must be used. Improvise using a rubber finger, baby bottle nipple, cosmetic sponge, or rubber ball. For example, the housing and tracheostoma adapter contained in the insufflation kit may be used by removing the catheter and plugging the attachment port or the housing may be used singly. If the stoma is relatively new, it is likely to shrink or change shape as further healing occurs. If occlusion continues to be a problem, a custom-molded tracheostoma housing may be considered.

5. The patient is now ready to learn to **coordinate breathing with stoma occlusion for speech** by inhaling, occluding the stoma, and producing either a sustained sound or words, such as counting. At the end of the production, the occlusion is released and a new breath is taken. Some laryngectomees master this instantly, whereas others require considerable practice using sentence drills of increasing length. When patients are successful with this, they are instructed to practice frequently throughout the day. As the patient becomes comfortable with the prosthesis and proficient in the act of occluding the stoma, speech usually becomes increasingly fluent and effortless.

6. **Refinement of tracheoesophageal voice** is accomplished using standard speech pathology treatment techniques.

   a. Encourage the laryngectomee to **speak with a minimum of effort** to achieve voice. The use of lowered resistance and larger diameter (20 French) prosthetics will assist the patient in achieving adequate airflow without unnecessary straining.

b. **Articulation drills** may facilitate improved intelligibility, particularly for patients who have had some involvement of the oral structures. The production of voiceless phonemes is particularly difficult for the alaryngeal speaker, but instruction in compensatory techniques, such as adjacent vowel lengthening, will result in increased listener recognition of the intended phoneme.

c. **Vocal pitch** can be consciously controlled to a degree in some alaryngeal speakers. Tracheoesophageal speech is typically lower in pitch than the average male laryngeal voice. The social consequences of the deep TE voice can be quite distressing for some female speakers. Although the mechanism of pitch variation is not well understood, the patient should be encouraged to use the most natural pitch that can be produced.

d. **Vocal loudness** is typically reduced in the alaryngeal speaker. The use of lowered resistance and larger diameter (20 French) prosthetics will result in increased airflow and assist the patient in achieving an optimal loudness level. The use of amplification, particularly when speaking before a group, is beneficial if adequate intensity cannot be achieved.

e. Improved speech naturalness can be achieved through exercises that emphasize **prosodic features**. Tracheoesophageal speakers are typically able to signal linguistic markers such as intonation, stress, juncture and duration. Phrasing should be consistent with the patient's pulmonary and phonatory abilities, as well as with grammatical conventions.

f. The **rate of speech** for TE speakers is generally slower than for laryngeal speakers. Attempts to increase the rate may result in reduced articulatory precision and loss of intelligibility.

g. If necessary, the patient can be instructed in the use of **compensatory strategies** to facilitate communication, such as maintaining proper eye contact, incorporating natural gestures, and reduction of background noise. Acceptability of TE speech can be increased by the elimination of mannerisms that draw unnecessary attention to the speaking act.

V. PATIENT INSTRUCTION

The importance of **patient teaching** cannot be overemphasized. Most minor complications with the tracheoesophageal puncture can be prevented or substantially minimized by developing the patient's (and/or caregiver's) understanding of the method of tracheoesophageal voice production, the use and care of the voice prosthesis, and the proper procedures to follow when problems arise. This should be taught in a slow, step-by-step process. In addition to demonstrations, ample opportunity for the patient to practice these new skills should be provided. Practice sessions should be held in a clean, well-lit area that contains a mirror and all necessary equipment. Written instructions should be provided to the patient for future reference.

A. General Instructions

The laryngectomee and caregiver should have a clear understanding of the **method of tracheoesophageal voice production** (see sample script in Appendix A). Even if this information was previously provided during preoperative counseling, a brief review will still be helpful as part of the training in tracheoesophageal voice production.

1. Begin by showing a diagram of the **anatomy before laryngectomy** (Figure 4–6). Indicate the location of important structures, such as the tongue, roof of mouth, trachea, larynx, and esophagus. Explain how the larynx functions as a valve to allow air movement between the lungs and mouth or nose for respiration, but closes to prevent aspiration during swallowing.

2. Provide a brief description of **normal speech production**. Explain how the closed vocal folds are set into vibration by exhaled air to achieve phonation, and how the sound is modified by the articulators to form the various speech sounds.

3. Using a diagram of the **anatomical changes** that result from laryngectomy (Figure 4–6), show how the windpipe ends at the stoma of the neck, the laryngeal sound source is removed, and there is no longer a connection between the windpipe and esophagus.

4. Explain the **sound source mechanism** of the pharyngoesophagus and the need for an air supply to set this tissue into vibration for voice production.

5. Using a diagram that illustrates the location of the voice prosthesis in the tracheoesophageal puncture tract, explain how the **tracheoesophageal puncture** (voice restoration) **procedure** has created a tunnel through the wall that separates the windpipe from the esophagus. This channel allows pulmonary air to move into the esophagus and drive the vibration of the PE segment.

6. Caution the patient that food, liquid, and saliva can leak through the puncture, and the prosthesis is used to prevent this. Demonstrate the **valving mechanism of a prosthesis** and show how it will be opened by pulmonary air when speech is attempted but will remain closed during swallowing to prevent aspiration. Emphasize that it is the vibration of the PE segment that is the sound source and not the prosthesis.

7. Most importantly, stress the role of the prosthesis in **keeping the puncture tract open**. In the absence of a prosthesis, dilating stent, or catheter, the puncture tract will close within a matter of hours and result in loss of tracheoesophageal voice. In the interim, aspiration of food, liquid, and saliva will occur. Closure of the puncture tract will require additional surgery to re-establish tracheoesophageal voice.

8. When the laryngectomee and/or caregiver demonstrate an adequate understanding of the method of tracheoesophageal voice restoration, instruction and practice in insertion of a **catheter or dilating stent** (Figure 6–3) should occur. The use of a mirror and a bright light directed toward the puncture site facilitate visualization and show the catheter correctly placed through the tract and not directed down the stoma. The patient must comprehend the importance of inserting the stent or catheter fully through the puncture tract, and the need to secure the device to the peristomal area firmly, in order to maintain the patency of the puncture.

9. The patient should receive instruction in **routine maintenance of the prosthesis**. The cleaning procedures will vary depending upon the type of device selected. Extended wear prostheses must be cleaned in situ using a flushing pipette (Figure 6–3) or supplied brush. The clinician should follow the manufacturer's instructions regarding the proper technique for a selected device. Care should be taken to avoid inserting clean-

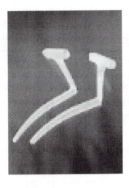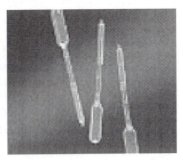

Figure 6–3. Left: Tracheoesophageal puncture dilator; **Right:** Flushing pipet. (Photos courtesy of InHealth.)

ing devices too deeply through the lumen of the prosthesis, because damage to the valving mechanism or to the esophagus may result.

B. Prosthesis Insertion and Removal

If the patient will be performing **self-insertion of the voice prosthesis**, the procedure should be thoroughly taught with ample opportunity for practice with the clinician until the requisite skills are mastered. The use of an extended wear prosthesis that is placed only by the physician or speech-language pathologist is recommended for patients who have difficulty learning the insertion technique, due to such factors such as poor vision, reduced manual dexterity, or cognitive decline. (See following section on Prosthesis Selection.)

1. **Practice sessions** are held in a clean, well-lit environment with a mirror and the necessary equipment, including forceps (tweezers), catheter or dilating stent, prosthesis insertion tool, tape, and surgical lubricant. The patient should be reminded to wash his or her hands prior to working around the stoma and puncture area.

2. Using written instructions (see example in Appendix A) as a guideline, the patient begins the process by **cleaning the stomal area** and removing any crusts around the prosthesis.

3. **Prepare the dilating stent/catheter** with a light film of surgical lubricant along the tip.

4. The patient is asked to swallow and then wait a few seconds. He or she is reminded to **refrain from swallowing** while the puncture tract is unstented.

5. The patient is instructed to **remove the prosthesis** by grasping the outer flange or strap close to the puncture site, and firmly pulling it forward.

6. The patient **places the dilating stent/catheter** into the puncture and secures it to the neck with adhesive tape.

7. **Clean and check the prosthesis** that is to be inserted according to the manufacturer's instructions. Check to make sure that the prosthesis valve is working and there is no sign of *candida* deposit (see section on Problem Solving and Appendix B).

8. Instruct the patient to **place the prosthesis on the insertion tool** and coat the tip with surgical lubricant.

9. The clinician talks the patient through the process as the stent/catheter is removed, **and the prosthesis is reinserted**, recognizing that coughing may occur and that several trials may be necessary. Some patients have particular difficulty in pushing the prosthesis through the puncture opening. The clinician must allow the patient to be successful in this task but not permit him or her to irritate the mucosa.

10. The patient is alerted to the **indications that the prosthesis is properly placed**. A "popping" sensation should be felt as the distal retention collar unfolds in the esophagus, and, while still attached to the insertion tool, the prosthesis should rotate freely in the tract.

11. When **proper placement is confirmed**, the strap is released from the insertion device and held with one hand as the insertion tool is removed from the voice prosthesis with a slight twist or rotating motion. The strap is secured to the skin with tape.

12. The laryngectomee should be provided with catalogs or other information for **ordering laryngectomy supplies**. No prescription is required for ordering supplies such as stoma covers, tape, and certain other accessories. However, for purchase of the first voice prosthesis, federal law requires that a pre-

scription from the physician or speech-language pathologist stating the type and size of the voice prosthesis must be on file with the manufacturer. Thereafter, patients who are capable of self-insertion of the prosthesis may contact the manufacturer directly to obtain replacement prostheses and accessories.

C. Problem Awareness and Emergency Instruction

The patient and caregiver will require thorough knowledge of the appropriate procedures to follow should an **emergency** arise. It is best to anticipate potential problems and have the patient be aware of the recommended steps to take, rather than hope that the patient will respond correctly by instinct alone. Occasionally a patient will deny or ignore a problem that could be easily solved if attended to on a timely basis, out of fear that the problem is a sign of disease recurrence. For example, a sudden loss of voice may be due to a prosthesis that is underfit or incorrectly placed, and can usually be remedied if addressed promptly. Delay in refitting the prosthesis correctly could result in closure of the puncture tract and necessitate additional surgery to restore the tracheoesophageal voice. The clinician should encourage open communication by instructing the patient to **contact the clinician promptly** if any problems arise, or if the patient is unsure about any aspect of the prosthesis or its functioning.

1. In case of **dislodgment of the voice prosthesis**, the patient should be prepared to place a dilating stentor catheter, or to replace the voice prosthesis. It is recommended that the patient carry either a small diameter (14–16 French) catheter or stent with him or her at all times. A stent or catheter can be used to maintain the puncture tract until the voice prosthesis can be properly replaced. Fortunately, this situation occurs less frequently since the advent of extended wear prostheses which have larger retention collars and are more resistant to dislodgment.

2. Patients should receive information concerning the course of action in the unlikely event of **aspiration of the voice prosthesis** into the stoma. The laryngectomee should not panic, because this may result in deep inhalations that draw the prosthesis further into the trachea. The patient should bend over at the waist and attempt to cough the prosthesis out of the trachea. If unsuccessful, emergency medical attention should be summoned for removal. The puncture should be stented immediately to avoid aspiration of esophageal contents into the lungs.

3. The most commonly occurring problem that a patient will encounter is **leakage through the prosthesis**. This is signaled by coughing at the instant of or just after a swallow. Patients should be aware that this problem is likely to occur and know the recommended procedures to follow. The specific course of action to be taken by the laryngectomee when leakage is observed will vary, dependent upon the underlying cause of the malfunction, type of prosthesis worn and whether the patient has been instructed in self-insertion of the prosthesis. To check for a leak, the patient is taught to illuminate the puncture with a bright light as a small sip of colored liquid is swallowed. If leaking is observed, prompt attention should be directed toward determining the cause and alleviating the problem to prevent continued aspiration and resultant pneumonia. (See Section IX on Problem Solving) Leakage through the prosthesis can be temporarily alleviated in some of the extended wear devices by use of a special accessory plug that seals the lumen of the device until the patient has the opportunity to return to the clinician for replacement.

4. Another common problem is **leaking around the prosthesis**. This is a condition that requires attention from the clinician to determine the underlying cause and course of action. The patient should be instructed to contact the clinician promptly in the event that leakage around the prosthesis occurs, because this condition rarely corrects itself and dislodgment of the prosthesis may result.

5. The **sudden loss of voice** after the laryngectomee has achieved satisfactory oral communication may be due to one of several factors. Most often it is related to a plugged or stuck prosthesis valve and can be remedied with proper cleaning of the device. (See following section on Maintenance of the Prosthesis.) Patients should be instructed to contact the clinician promptly if the voice does not return to its usual quality after cleaning of the device, because this may be an indication of closure of the puncture tract or changes in the vibratory characteristics of the PE segment.

6. The patient should be instructed to return to the clinician promptly for **prosthesis refitting** if it appears that the prosthesis length is no longer appropriate. A prosthesis that is too long may piston in the puncture and cause dilation of the tract, resulting in leakage around the prosthesis and eventual dis-

lodgment. Reduction of the available airway may also result from a prosthesis that is too long. A prosthesis that may be too short and appears to be receding into the puncture may result in loss of the puncture tract, necessitating further surgery to restore the voice.

7. The laryngectomee should be alerted to watch for signs of **redness, irritation, or other tissue changes** that may signal infection, improper healing of the tracheoesophageal puncture tract, or inflammatory reaction. The patient should return to the clinician for evaluation if any of these occur.

8. It is helpful to provide every laryngectomee with an **emergency card** that can be carried in the wallet or shirt pocket at all times. The card should contain information on first aid for neck breathers, a concise description of tracheoesophageal puncture, and clinician contact information. Emergency medical personnel typically have little if any training in rescue breathing for laryngectomees and may inadvertently attempt to administer oxygen transorally or transnasally when every second counts. Basic information concerning the voice prosthesis can assist medical professionals in providing appropriate treatment that does not compromise the function of the tracheoesophageal puncture should the patient be unable to explain the method of TEP speech adequately. Bracelets and necklaces containing emergency medical information are also available commercially and should at least contain the information that the individual is a "neck breather."

VI. PROSTHESIS SELECTION

A. Concerns and Considerations

As technology and our understanding of the mechanism of tracheoesophageal voice have advanced, **a variety of prostheses have become available**. Each device has distinct advantages and disadvantages, and there is no single prosthesis that meets the needs of all patients. Furthermore, the specific requirements of an individual patient may change over time, and the prosthesis that is selected initially may not be appropriate for long-term use. The clinician, in consultation with the laryngectomee, must weigh several factors to determine which device will offer the optimum benefit for a specific individual.

The **primary concerns in selecting the prosthesis** type are to maintain the patency of the puncture tract and promote healthy tissue of the tracheoesophageal wall.

1. A 16 French duckbill style is often selected for the **initial fitting of the voice prosthesis** and when there is a concern for edema of the tracheoesophageal wall, as may occur during radiotherapy. The smaller diameter is preferable until the puncture site heals. The contour of the distal tip permits smooth insertion, and its slightly increased extension into the esophagus helps guard against underfitting and stenosis of the esophageal side of the puncture if edema occurs.

2. If the **tissue of the tracheoesophageal wall** has been heavily radiated or is weakened due to poorly controlled diabetes, nutritional imbalance, or other medical factors, a 16 French prosthesis made of soft silicone should be selected, because the larger, stiffer devices may cause irritation and/or dilation of the tract.

3. The **thickness of the tracheoesophageal party wall** may limit the choice of prosthetic devices, because some styles are not manufactured in extremely short or long lengths.

4. For patients with a **narrowed esophagus**, a duckbill style prosthesis may impinge on the posterior esophageal wall. This may prevent the prosthesis valve from opening, resulting in poor vocal quality, or alternately, it may cause the prosthesis to remain in the open position, resulting in leakage through the prosthesis.

5. When all requirements have been met to maintain the patency of the puncture tract and ensure the viability of the tracheoesophageal tissue, the clinician should consider the **aerodynamic characteristics** that will promote a satisfactory vocal quality with a minimum of effort. The aerodynamic specifications of each device are available from the manufacturer so that accurate comparisons can be made. Some general guidelines follow.

   a. The duckbill type devices typically have a **higher resistance to airflow** than most of the hinged or ball valve devices, resulting in a voice of lower volume. However, the increased resistance may be beneficial for patients who experience excessive gas that is due to the inhalation of air through a prosthesis of lower resistance during quiet respiration.

b. The hinged and ball type valved prostheses (sometimes marketed as "low pressure" prostheses) typically have a **lower resistance to airflow** and generally result in a louder vocal volume and less respiratory effort.

c. The larger (20 French) diameter devices result in **greater airflow** through the puncture tract, requiring less respiratory effort and resulting in an increased phonatory volume.

6. If there are any concerns regarding **the patient's ability to care for the device**, an extended wear prosthesis should be selected. These prostheses are typically less likely to dislodge accidentally due to the design of the esophageal retention collar and they require infrequent changes by the speech-language pathologist or physician, reducing the patient's responsibility for maintaining the device.

7. When there is limited **availability of medical support services** in the patient's community, an extended wear device that can only be replaced by a physician or speech-language pathologist may represent a poor choice of prosthesis. Devices that are less commonly used, such as some of the imported prostheses, are contraindicated for patients who travel extensively and may require urgent support services while away from home.

8. The **ease of insertion** is maximal for the duckbill style prostheses, owing to the rounded distal tip. The trauma of insertion can be reduced for some of the hinged valve prostheses, which have a blunt tip, by use of a gelatin capsule system that encases the esophageal retention collar and contours the distal tip. The "retrograde insertion" required for some of the extended wear devices, by which the prosthesis is drawn through the oropharynx and into the puncture tract, can be uncomfortable for many patients, necessitating the use of topical anesthesia to reduce gagging. This placement technique is useful however, when there is a separation of the tracheoesophageal party wall and a concern that the prosthesis is not completely through the puncture tract when using the standard "front-loading" insertion technique.

9. In some circumstances, **economic factors** may influence the choice of prosthesis. In calculating the total cost, the clinician will need to consider the retail price of the prosthesis, as well as the typical longevity of each device.

VII. THE TRACHEOSTOMA VALVE

The **tracheostoma valve** eliminates the need for digital occlusion of the stoma for speech production. Patients must be selected and fitted with the valve (Figure 6–4).

A. Description

The **design of the valve** allows quiet breathing to be unimpeded. A thin diaphragm responds to the natural increase in air pressure for speech by closing and diverting air through the prosthesis. The valve automatically reopens when the air pressure diminishes at the end of the expiration/utterance. There is a flexible housing or collar (similar to that used in the insufflation test) which is sealed externally to the peristomal skin with adhesives. A tight seal is essential for the valve to function. Alternately, the patient is fitted with a type of laryngectomy tube housing, sometimes referred to as a "stoma button," that resides in the stoma and accommodates the tracheostoma valve. Should these attachment methods prove unsatisfactory, the patient can be fitted for a custom housing made of prosthodontic materials. The valve is inserted into one of these applied housings and can be quickly removed, if necessary, leaving the housing in place.

B. Patient Selection

Patients with significant respiratory problems may not be good candidates for use of the valve. Similarly, patients who experience excessive mucous discharge and secretions find the valve problematic. The benefits of "hands-free" speech and improved hygiene suggest that all patients should be considered for a trial with the valve to determine its efficacy for them.

1. Patients should be **speaking effectively using digital stoma occlusion** and the prosthesis should be functioning properly for a minimum of 1 month before the tracheostoma valve is attempted. This will ensure that the patient has learned efficient respiratory control for tracheoesophageal speech before

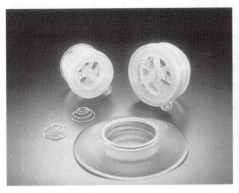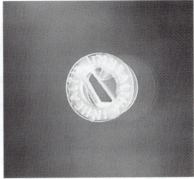

Figure 6–4. Tracheostoma valves. Left: Bivona. (Photo courtesy of Bivona.) **Right:** In-Health. (Photo courtesy of InHealth.)

adding the additional respiratory maneuvers that are required for activating the tracheostoma valve.

2. Patients should be fully informed about the **nature of the valve and how it works.** They should be given the opportunity to examine the components of the valve and taught how to insert the valve and remove it from the housing. They should be allowed to practice this prior to affixing the housing to the neck.

C. Valve Placement

Attachment of an external housing device with adhesives requires a meticulous technique to ensure a proper seal. The laryngectomee should be taught in a step-by-step fashion in a well-lit room while seated in front of a mirror. Several housing types of various sizes and shapes are currently available to accommodate the variability of stomal configurations. One system features a reusable plastic disc that is affixed using double-sided tape and/or foam discs in conjunction with a liquid skin adhesive. Other housings come with a pre-applied adhesive and are for one-time use. The manufacturers' specific instructions for attachment of the housing devices should be followed closely to ensure maximum adherence. Alternately a stoma button may be adapted for use with the valve. General guidelines follow.

1. The **peristomal area** should be clean and dry. There are several skin barrier products (e.g., Shield Skin® or Skin-Prep™) available to help cleanse the skin thoroughly and increase adherence of the housing device. Care should be taken to

avoid dripping of these products into the stoma. The strap on the non-extended-wear prostheses may be shortened by approximately ¼ inch prior to insertion. If the strap contains a hole for locking it on to the insertion tool, it should not be cut beyond this point.

2. If a **liquid adhesive** is used, it should be spread thinly around the stoma corresponding to the size of the housing. Extra attention should be given to suture lines, skin folds, and other irregularities of the peristomal area, because this is typically where the seal will break. Care should be taken to avoid getting any adhesive into the stoma. The adhesive should be allowed to dry before affixing the housing. Both sides of the strap of the non-extended-wear prostheses should be prepared with a small amount of adhesive, and the strap should be pressed against the skin using a blunt instrument to avoid finger contact with the adhesive.

3. If necessary, the **housing is prepared** with the double-sided tape disc and/or foam disc. The use of the foam disc can help counteract the irregularity of the peristomal area. Finger and surface contact with the adhesive discs, resulting in loss of adherence, can be avoided by placing the index finger inside the opening of the housing and the thumb on the outside edge. It is necessary to seal the contact between the housing and the discs manually or with the use of a blunt-ended instrument firmly in order to remove all air bubbles.

4. The **housing is placed** up to the designated area around the stoma, ideally with the opening of the housing slightly below the upper rim of the stoma. Slight neck extension will facilitate flattening of the peristomal area as the housing is applied.

5. Beginning with problem areas such as suture lines and skin folds, the **housing is pressed to the neck**, bending the flexible housing to fit the contour of the neck, and working from the inner area toward the edges to ensure a tight seal.

6. As an alternative to the external housings, the tracheostoma valve can be placed in a **stoma button** (Barton-Mayo tracheostoma button), a small device resembling a very short laryngectomy tube worn in the trachea. The use of the button eliminates the need for potentially irritating skin adhesives.

a. To **insert the stoma button**, a light film of olive oil or surgical lubricant is placed on the end that enters the stoma. The button is flattened then folded in half and placed into the stoma. As it is released, it will open and conform to the shape of the stoma.

b. To allow the **passage of expired air into the prosthesis**, a small window must be cut into the posterior wall of the button, corresponding to the location of the prosthesis inlet.

c. The **button can be removed** by grasping one side and pulling toward the other side. Pulling the device straight forward from the stoma will cause irritation of the tracheal tissue.

7. The **tracheostoma valve is inserted** into the housing while placing one hand on the housing to hold it in place. To insert the valve, it should be grasped by the edge (not by the bar that goes across the top; that is meant to keep clothing away from the valve). Insert the lower edge of the valve (as you are holding it) into the bottom of the housing opening, and push down gently to stretch the opening slightly downward. Roll the valve in toward the top of the opening, like a door on a hinge, and push it inward. It should pop into place using this maneuver, but may take some practice to learn to do easily. With the valve in place, the patient should be instructed to sit quietly for a short time to be reassured that breathing is unimpaired.

8. The patient is then instructed to **produce easy speech** starting with a quick exhalation to close the valve. The exhaled air pressure must be sufficient to close the valve. If the valve seal is firm, the valve diaphragm will be heard to close and speech will be produced. If the diaphragm does not close, make certain that sufficient air pressure is being exerted and that air is not leaking around the housing. Allow several trials.

9. Tracheostoma valves are supplied in one of several different **closure sensitivities**, or they come with an adjustment mechanism to tailor the closure sensitivity in relation to the air pressure demands of the task. The ideal valve sensitivity allows for easy quiet breathing, minimal effort for valve closure during speech, and a lack of inadvertent spontaneous closure during normal physical activity. A trial and error process attempting various speech tasks and physical activities such as walking or stair climbing may be necessary to determine the appropriate sensitivity.

10. The **valve is removed** by stabilizing the housing against the neck with one hand while grasping the edge of the valve with the other hand and pulling it open like a hinged door from one side. The valve should not be grasped or pulled by the bar.

   a. When the onset of a **cough** is sensed, the valve should be removed leaving the housing in place. Secretions should be thoroughly wiped from inside the stoma and around the housing prior to reinserting the valve.

   b. The valve should not be worn during **sleep**. The housing should not be left on for longer periods than recommended by the manufacturers because the peristomal skin may become irritated.

11. After removing the housing, the **skin should be cleaned** with warm water and soap. Adhesive residue can be easily removed by the use of adhesive remover products available from the prosthesis manufacturer. If using a reusable housing, the adhesive disc will need to be removed and the housing cleaned according to the manufacturer's instructions.

D. Valve Use

1. As with the prosthesis, the **patient must be instructed** in affixing the housing and inserting the valve. The latter is particularly important because of the need to remove the valve during or after coughing, or at any other time that it may require cleaning. (See Appendix A for sample patient handout.)

2. Patients may need **short-term therapy** to learn to use the valve effectively. Attention should be given to easy speech production with minimal strain, length of utterances consistent with pulmonary air supply, appropriate phrasing, and good coordination of exhalation and speech.

3. It takes practice for most laryngectomees to be successful with the hands-free tracheostoma valves. The use of **minimum respiratory effort** is critical to reducing the "back pressure" that contributes to the premature loss of the seal. With repeated applications, the likely location of adhesive seal failures will become obvious. Special attention should be focused on these areas when applying the adhesives. If the problem persists, the need for additional adjustments to the housing should be considered.

VIII. TRACHEOESOPHAGEAL PUNCTURE IN EXTENDED RECONSTRUCTIONS

As surgical reconstructive techniques of the pharyngoesophagus have advanced (see Chapter 8), it has become possible for patients to be considered for tracheoesophageal voice restoration. A careful assessment of candidacy should be made, including insufflation testing, and the patient should be counseled regarding realistic expectations for vocal function.

A. Types of Reconstructions

1. Reconstruction of partial pharyngeal defects with a **pectoralis major myocutaneous flap** usually results in adequate vocal quality, and puncture may be possible at the time of laryngectomy.

2. Reconstruction of more extensive pharyngeal defects with a **tubed radial forearm flap** will also usually provide a satisfactory voice with only slight reductions in vocal characteristics compared to standard TE speakers. Prosthetic rehabilitation is typically done as a secondary procedure after adequate healing of the free tissue transfer has occurred.

3. The use of a **free jejunal tissue transfer** for replacement of the entire pharynx typically results in a fair voice. Frequently the voice sounds "wet" due to continuous production of secretions and the vibratory function may be hindered by the autonomous peristalsis of the jejunal segment. The use of digital pressure, pressure bands, and head turning may aid in establishing a more satisfactory vibration (Kelly & Huff, 1980). The laryngectomee with jejunal reconstruction should be eating well and respond favorably to air insufflation to be considered for voice restoration.

4. A **gastric transposition (pull-up)** procedure is performed for total laryngopharyngectomy with total esophagectomy. The vocal quality may vary from tight and strained to loose and wet with this procedure. Satisfactory voice can usually be obtained with careful problem solving. As with the free tissue transfer procedures, voice restoration is usually delayed until adequate healing is complete.

5. In **total laryngectomy with total glossectomy**, various surgical reconstructive techniques will be employed simultane-

ously to fill the extensive tissue defects. The emphasis is typically on restoration of the oral and pharyngeal cavities to allow oral nutrition. Successful speech rehabilitation has been achieved for a limited number of patients. Tracheoesophageal voice restoration is aided by a prosthetic tongue or palatal lowering device. Intelligibility can be significantly compromised requiring extensive speech rehabilitation.

IX. PROBLEM SOLVING

Problem areas and their solutions have been identified as experience with this method of voice restoration has grown. The most commonly occurring problems, potential causative factors, and suggested possible solutions are summarized in Appendix B.

A. General Considerations

Aphonia or effortful phonation may be due to several causes. Some warrant urgent attention by the clinician. Careful problem solving will usually determine the nature of the aphonia or effortful voice and suggest possible solutions.

1. The first level of determination should be to ascertain whether the aphonia is due to a **problem with the prosthesis or with the patient's ability** to vibrate the pharyngoesophageal segment. This is done with the open-tract test (see the previous Procedure for Fitting section) in which the prosthesis is removed momentarily and the patient attempts to phonate while the clinician performs the stoma occlusion. If voice improves significantly while phonating with an open tract, one can assume that the vibratory segment is functioning and the problem, therefore, is either with the prosthesis, or the patient's technique of stoma occlusion.

2. Aphonia or a strained voice can be caused by **problems with the prosthesis** that prohibit the opening of the valve and the free flow of air through the lumen.

3. If the patient has been fitted with an extended wear voice prosthesis that cannot be re-inserted because the strap has been removed, the clinician may wish to forego the open tract test and attempt to **determine the nature of the problem in situ.** If such conservative procedures fail to establish the nature of the problem, the open tract test should then be attempted with

the understanding that the prosthesis will need to be replaced with a new device.

B. Specific Problems

1. A **prosthesis that is too long** (especially if a duckbill type) may impale the posterior wall of the esophagus and fail to open for phonation. Esophageal irritation will result if the prosthesis is not promptly replaced.

2. **Crusting** of mucus, saliva, or food particles may cause the valve to remain in the closed position. This is easily remedied by cleaning the voice prosthesis in situ.

3. Changing to a different style of prosthesis (low pressure or larger diameter) will correct aphonia that is due to the use of a **prosthesis with excessive resistance**.

4. If the prosthesis has been inserted with a **gelatin capsule**, it is necessary to wait approximately 4–5 minutes for it to dissolve before voicing can be expected.

5. A **prosthesis that is too short or not fully inserted** is typically indicated by a deteriorating vocal ability that begins one hour to several days after the prosthesis has been placed. Occasionally, an incorrectly inserted prosthesis will result in the creation of a false puncture tract which does not extend through the common tracheoesophageal wall into the esophagus. A prosthesis that is too short or incorrectly inserted can be misdiagnosed easily, because the prosthesis may be extruding into the stoma, giving the false impression that the prosthesis is too long, and suggesting that downsizing of the prosthesis is the solution. The situation is further complicated by problems in measuring the tract, because the esophageal end of the puncture will have started to stenose, making it difficult to insert the measuring device fully. Failure to correct this problem promptly by proper stenting of the puncture will result in closure of the tract and necessitate surgical intervention to re-establish the tracheoesophageal puncture.

   a. If this problem is suspected, the **correct placement of the prosthesis can be verified** by one of two methods. If the prosthesis is radiopaque, an x-ray of the cervical region may be helpful in making the determination. Alternately, flexible endoscopy of the pharyngoesophageal (see Appendix B for a description of this method) may reveal correct placement of the prosthesis (Figure 6–5).

b. If correct placement cannot be determined with certainty using either of these methods, the clinician should remove the prosthesis and place a dilating catheter. **The primary concern must always be for fully maintaining the puncture tract.** If the esophageal end of the puncture has begun to stenose, it may be difficult to insert a catheter of a diameter equal to that of the prosthesis. In this situation, begin with a small catheter (10 or 12 French) and serially dilate until a catheter one size larger than the prosthesis diameter can be passed through the tract. This catheter should remain in place for a minimum of 24 hours to dilate the tract fully before re measurement and prosthesis placement are attempted.

c. In the event that the smallest available catheter (8–10 French) cannot be inserted fully through the tract, the patient should attempt to swallow very small sips of water while the puncture is unstented. The presence of a small leak during the swallow will ascertain that the puncture is still viable. The patient should be **referred to the physician** for immediate attempt to salvage the puncture. The absence of a leak through the unstented puncture suggests that the esophageal end of the puncture has closed. In this case, the puncture should remain unstented and the patient should be referred to the physician. Re puncture may be performed in approximately 4–6 weeks after the tract has fully closed.

6. Should aphonia or strained vocal quality persist during the open tract test, the clinician should further **evaluate the vibratory capabilities of the pharyngoesohageal segment**. Vibratory function of the pharyngoesophageal segment is dependent on tissue elasticity and aerodynamic driving forces.

7. **Reduced pulmonary support** for speech production is usually indicated by low volume productions of short duration. The use of a low resistance prosthesis type can help to minimize the effects of this condition.

8. **Edema** of the pharyngoesophagus, which may occur with radiation, esophageal dilations, or immediately postpuncture,

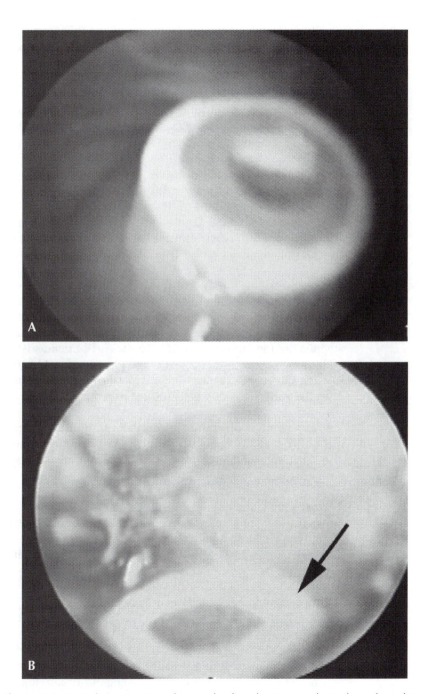

Figure 6–5. A: Endoscopic view of correctly placed voice prosthesis through tracheo-esophageal wall and into esophagus. **B:** Voice prosthesis not placed through the tracheoesophageal wall appears as a circular shadow under endoscopic evaluation.

will reduce the vibratory capabilities of the PE segment. If edema is suspected at the time of fitting, the catheter should be replaced for several days or weeks until it subsides.

9. **Pharyngeal constrictor hypertonicity** or spasm can occur as a response to air insufflation of the esophagus. This condition can usually be managed successfully by pharyngeal constrictor myotomy or chemodenervation with botulinum toxin injections.

10. **Forceful stoma occlusion** can result in excessive pressure against the esophagus that restricts the free flow of air across the vibratory segment. Light digital occlusion or the use of the hands-free tracheostoma valve are the recommended solutions.

11. **Excessively low pitch** can be due to a loose or hypotonic segment. This condition occurs most frequently when there has been extended reconstruction of the pharyngoesophagus. External digital pressure, head turning, or a pressure band applied to the vibratory area of the neck will often assist in obtaining the requisite contact of the PE walls for vibratory activity. Therapy exercises directed toward consciously altering the vocal pitch may benefit some patients.

12. **Strained, high pitch** may be an indication of pharyngeal constrictor hypertonicity or spasm. In some cases, an attempt to lower vocal pitch and/or reduce vocal effort may result in improvement.

13. **Short phrases** may be the result of pharyngeal constrictor hypertonicity or of excessive effort. It is necessary first to rule out or address hypertonicity, and to attempt the use of larger diameter and low resistance prosthetics. Then respiratory effort should be retrained.

14. **Wet, gurgly vocal quality** is usually due to pooling of liquids or secretions in the pharynx above the PE segment. The patient should be encouraged to swallow frequently or perform a throat clearing maneuver by inhaling moderately, occluding the stoma, then exhaling steadily while prolonging a "hum-m-m" sound. Sipping small amounts of warm liquids may also help to clear these secretions. In severe cases, the patient should be assessed by the surgeon for the presence of a diverticulum.

15. **The unexplained loss of vibratory capability** of the PE segment following a period of successful voice restoration should be promptly evaluated by the physician to rule out the possibility of disease recurrence.

C. Leakage

The most commonly occurring problem is **leakage through or around the prosthesis**. This is signaled by coughing during swallowing or staining of the stoma cover. To check for a leak, the puncture is illuminated with a bright light as a small sip of colored liquid is swallowed. If leaking is observed, prompt attention should be directed toward determining the cause and alleviating the problem to prevent continued aspiration and resultant pneumonia.

1. **Leakage through the prosthesis** will occur due to valve deterioration. The typical device life is from 2 to 4 months, but it will be shortened by colonization of *candida* or other organisms on the prosthesis (see below). Other causes of leakage through the prosthesis are discussed below.

   a. **Deposits of *candida*** on the silicone prosthesis have been associated with premature valve failure due to leakage through the prosthesis and with difficulty producing sound due to increased resistance of the device. Additionally, the prosthesis may be colonized with several varieties of bacteria. Some laryngectomees seem to have a low *candida* presence, whereas others may have a predilection for an extended period. Chemotherapy and radiation treatment are factors that can promote an environment that is favorable for fungal growth. For patients who replace the voice prosthesis independently, one solution would be to have multiple prostheses, wearing one of the prostheses for 1 to 3 days and soaking the alternate prostheses in hydrogen peroxide. For the extended wear devices, the use of nystatin mouthwash or amphotericin lozenges will assist in the control of *candida*. It is essential, however, that the nystatin mouthwash be held in the mouth for approximately 3–4 minutes for it to be effective. Some of the extended wear prostheses (Provox®, Provox2®, and Voice Master®) are impregnated with an anti-*candida* treatment of the valving mechanism to extend device life. It is recommended that the extended wear prosthetics be replaced a minimum of every 6 months, due to colonization along the prosthesis shaft that may result in dilation of the puncture tract.

b. The valving mechanism may fail to close properly if **the esophageal end is impaled against the posterior wall** of the esophagus (especially the duckbill style). This is easily remedied by using the hinged-type prosthesis of an appropriate length.

c. Temporary leakage may also be caused by crusting of secretions or food, or if the prosthesis is deformed during the insertion process.

d. A less common cause of leakage of the low resistance prostheses is due **to movement of the hinged valve in response to changing air pressures** associated with respiration or swallowing. The use of a higher resistance valving mechanism will usually correct the problem.

2. **Leakage around the prosthesis** is usually due to dilation of the puncture tract and requires prompt attention to prevent potential dislodgment of the prosthesis. Tract dilation can be the result of several conditions.

a. Placement of a **voice prosthesis** that is too long will cause it to piston in the tract and irritate the tissue. The prosthesis should be replaced with one of appropriate length.

b. The use of the **stiff silicone** found in some extended wear devices can result in tract dilation. This can usually be reversed by use of the softer silicone devices.

c. **Plaque deposits** on the exterior shaft of the extended wear prostheses will enlarge the outside diameter of the device and cause a slow dilation of the tract over time. Following prosthesis replacement, leakage around the new device may occur until the tract conforms to the standard prosthesis diameter. This can be prevented by more frequent changing of the prosthesis, usually every 6 months.

d. Leakage may also occur if the **integrity of the tracheoesophageal wall** is compromised due to high-dose radiation, diabetes, or other medical conditions. In these circumstances, the tract should be allowed to shrink down around a small, soft catheter (14–16 French) for 3–4 weeks, and then a prosthesis of soft silicone that has a sufficiently large retention collar should be placed.

e. Leakage around the prosthesis may also be an indicator of **local disease recurrence** which results in a loss of tissue elasticity. The benefits of maintaining the puncture in the setting of malignant disease should be carefully considered.

f. Directing the stenting catheter upward in the pharyngoesophagus at the time of tracheoesophageal puncture may cause the puncture to assume a keyhole configuration as it heals. This can be avoided by directing the stenting catheter downward into the esophagus.

g. Infrequently, puncture dilation will not respond to the previous conservative treatment measures. In the case of **unrelenting dilation**, the puncture should be allowed to stenose completely using the procedure described below (see Section on Failed Cases), or it should be closed surgically. It may be necessary for the surgeon to reconstruct the tracheoesophageal wall using a myocutaneous flap before repuncture is considered.

D. Other Problems

1. Patients undergoing **radiation therapy** after being fitted with a prosthesis may find a temporary disruption in their ability to speak during the course of radiotherapy because of swelling and inflammation of the tissues. Speech should return naturally as those problems resolve. However, as edema of the tracheoesophageal common wall may occur, the length of the voice prosthesis may become inadequate to maintain the puncture tract fully. The clinician should alert patients to this potential complication and instruct them to return to the clinician at the first indication that the prosthesis may be underfit (e.g., voice loss, strained voice, prosthesis retraction into the puncture, or prosthesis extrusion). Laryngectomees who undergo tracheoesophageal voice restoration after radiation may experience aphonia or a strained vocal quality initially until edema subsides. This may continue for a few months after completion of radiotherapy. It is important to distinguish this type of aphonia from pharyngeal constrictor spasm, because the treatments are different for the two conditions (see previous section on Aphonia).

2. Granulation tissue formation may occur as a result of an inflammatory foreign body reaction to the prosthesis, tissue trauma related to the insertion procedure, particularly in prostheses that are changed infrequently, and in the presence of *candida.* The solution to this problem is more frequent removal using a gentle technique, and proper cleaning of the prosthesis with measures to control *candida* overgrowth. Cauterization or surgical excision of the granulation may be required. In the presence of granulation tissue, prosthesis insertion trauma can be reduced by dilating the tract two sizes larger than the prosthesis, using a surgical lubricant, and use of a gelatin capsule system for the blunt-tipped prostheses.

3. The presence of the TEP may induce an inflammatory reaction that has been linked to a low incidence of **tracheostomal stenosis**, resulting in microstoma. This can be managed successfully through the use of a silicone laryngectomy tube, but it may require surgical stomal revision if the situation advances to the degree that the airway is compromised.

4. **Prolapse of the esophageal mucosa** through the puncture tract occurs in a small number of cases, complicating prosthesis insertion. This can be managed by thorough dilation of the puncture two sizes larger than the prosthesis that is to be placed.

5. **Difficult or painful insertion** will occur if the puncture tract has not been fully dilated or is beginning to stenose. Proper dilation will ease the insertion procedure and help to ensure correct placement of the device. The use of a surgical lubricant and a gelatin capsule system will also reduce insertion trauma.

6. Painful insertion is sometimes associated with **gastroesophageal reflux**, and an anti-reflux protocol will reduce this difficulty.

7. In a small number of patients, the attempted removal and/or placement of a catheter, stent, or prosthesis will stimulate **excessive coughing and regurgitation**. If this occurs, the puncture should be stented immediately to prevent soiling of the trachea. The use of topical anesthesia to the stoma and oropharynx may reduce this tendency on subsequent insertion attempts.

8. **The location of the puncture** may compromise the ease of insertion. Neck extension, lifting any overlapping peristomal

skin, and reclining the patient can be helpful if the puncture tract is difficult to visualize. Slow, careful insertion of a catheter with attention to the tactile sensations will help determine the angle of a puncture tract. A puncture that is angled upward can sometimes be redirected by placing a catheter that is angled downward to the esophagus for several days. Stoma revision or repuncture may be necessary in extreme cases.

9. **Excess gastric air** is experienced by a small number of laryngectomees and causes discomfort and may interfere with fluent speech.

10. **Pharyngoesophageal stricture** (scar formation) may cause narrowing to the extent that food transit and the flow of air through the pharyngoesophagus are impeded. Air exiting the prosthesis will be forced to the stomach. Treatment is by mechanical dilation of the pharyngoesophagus or surgical revision.

11. **Pharyngeal constrictor hypertonicity** will also restrict the egress of tracheoesophageal air and force it into the stomach. Pharyngeal constrictor myotomy or chemical denervation with botulinum toxin to manage the hypertonicity will result in decreased phonatory effort as well as a decrease in excess gastric air.

12. **Movement of the hinged valve in response to changing air pressures** associated with respiration or swallowing can result in the inhalation of air through the prosthesis and into the esophagus. The use of a higher resistance valving mechanism will usually correct the problem.

13. A **hypotonic PE segment** may also result in the inhalation of air through the mouth and nose with each respiratory cycle. This is typically associated with weak breathy phonation. The use of a pressure band worn around the neck may help to correct this problem.

14. **Short duration of the tracheostoma valve seal** is a common problem that requires careful problem solving by the clinician and determination on the part of the laryngectomee. The benefits of "hands-free" speech and improved hygiene suggest that a concerted effort be made to ensure success with this device.

15. **Excessive "back pressure"** against the tracheostoma housing is caused by increased phonatory effort. The pressure can be assessed by using a manometer during speech to provide feedback to the patient. A conscious reduction in phonatory loudness and respiratory effort, coupled with the use of lowered resistance or larger diameter (20 French) prostheses are effective in reducing the back pressure.

16. **Inattention to a meticulous technique** when applying adhesives and attaching the housing will result in a poor seal. The skin should be clean and dry, liquid adhesives should be allowed to set for the recommended times, and air bubbles should be eliminated. Retraining in the proper techniques or the use of self-adhering housings may be helpful.

17. **An irregular peristomal area** represents a challenge for the attachment of the housing device. The solution may lie in the use of the larger, self-adhering housings, the use of skin-barrier products, and neck extension to smooth the surface prior to attachment.

18. Prior to coughing, the tracheostoma valve should be removed and **stomal secretions** should be carefully wiped from the inside surface of the housing chimney. Excessive secretions can be effectively reduced by the use of heat-moisture exchange systems or with prescription medications.

19. The use of a **Barton-Mayo button or a custom fabricated housing device** (made by a prosthodontist) should be considered if the standard housing devices cannot be used successfully.

X. TRACHEOESOPHAGEAL PUNCTURE FAILURE

Estimates of successful TEP voice restoration range from 85–95%. Failed voice restoration can be due to a number of reasons. Many are preventable.

A. Causes of TEP Failure

1. The most common cause of TEP failure is due to **unplanned closure of the puncture tract**. This is almost always preven-

table if the prosthesis has been properly fitted and the patient (and/or caregiver) has received thorough instruction in emergency precautions, for example placement of a stenting catheter.

2. **Unrelenting dilation of the puncture tract** can often be prevented by careful selection of appropriate stenting devices and prosthetics. However, in a small number of cases, the dilation continues to progress despite all efforts to contain it. In these cases, the puncture should be allowed to stenose (see discussion below on Planned Closure) or be closed surgically. The decision to repuncture at a later date should be made cautiously, with consideration given to contributing conditions, such as diabetes or high dose radiation.

3. **Failure to develop the necessary skills** for satisfactory voice production and maintenance of the voice prosthesis may be due to cognitive or medical conditions that preclude learning. This can usually be avoided by careful selection of candidates for the procedure.

4. **Local disease recurrence** may limit the vibratory characteristics of the PE segment or result in unmanageable dilation of the puncture due to a loss of tissue elasticity. The presence of distant malignant disease does not preclude successful voice restoration.

5. **Reduced intelligibility or poor vocal quality** is usually the result of extensive reconstruction or may be due to other confounding medical conditions. Careful attention to screening of TEP candidates will avoid this problem.

6. TEP failures related to **patient preference** for other methods of alaryngeal communication can be minimized by frank discussions with the patient regarding communication options and expected outcomes prior to puncture.

7. **Planned closure of the TE puncture tract** is accomplished in graduated steps to prevent unwanted complications, for example, aspiration pneumonia. The puncture should be stented with a soft catheter that is one size smaller on successive nights until a size 8 French is reached. Care should be taken that the catheter is securely affixed to the neck and will not dislodge during sleep. Downsizing the catheter before retiring is advisable due to the decreased frequency of swal-

lowing during sleep. When the puncture has been successfully downsized, the final catheter should be removed, and the puncture should be checked for leaks by swallowing a small sip of liquid. If only a small leak is present, the catheter can be left out and the puncture allowed to close spontaneously. Until closure is complete, the patient should mix liquids with solids to reduce the chance of aspiration through the puncture. If the fistula fails to close, cauterization or a Z-plasty surgical technique may be employed by the physician to close the puncture.

XI. NEW DEVELOPMENTS

Tracheoesophageal puncture has gained worldwide acceptance as a method of alaryngeal voice restoration since its inception in the late 1970s. As the technology advances and experience with this procedure increases, there will continue to be improvements in surgical techniques and prosthesis design. Research is now directed toward understanding the physiologic mechanism of pharyngoesophageal sound production. This will result in improved methods of surgical reconstruction that maximize phonatory capabilities without sacrificing cancer control. Prosthesis design will focus on meeting the aerodynamic requirements for effortless speech production and incorporating extended wear features that will minimize the maintenance required by the laryngectomee. An improved global communication network has already resulted in the increasingly free exchange of information regarding problem-solving methodologies. At the same time, trends toward managed care reimbursement for health expenses and a movement against specialization place additional demands on health care professionals to provide high quality services of demonstrated efficacy to the alaryngeal speaker. Other changes are certain, and the speech-language pathologist must stay abreast of new developments to provide state-of-the-art services to laryngectomized persons.

CHAPTER

7

Characteristics of Alaryngeal and Glossectomy Speech

The intent of this chapter is to describe some of the acoustical, physiological, and perceptual characteristics of alaryngeal speech. Information is presented that may assist clinicians who work with laryngectomees. In addition, some data drawn from the literature are presented to provide the clinician with a readily available source of information against which to compare a patient's performance. Finally, clinicians are strongly encouraged to collect pertinent, objective data about their patients to document and monitor progress and to evaluate specific therapeutic strategies.

I. ACOUSTIC CHARACTERISTICS

A. Fundamental Frequency (F_0)

1. Most **mechanical speech aids** are electronic and have a manually adjustable fundamental frequency (see Figure 7–1A). These are typically set to a low pitch for a male voice (about 100 Hz) and, where possible, to a higher value for a female voice (about 200 Hz). Some have a variable frequency adjustment. Because F_0 is determined by the electronic design of the specific instrument, little data have been reported on the F_0 characteristics of speech produced with the electrolarynx.

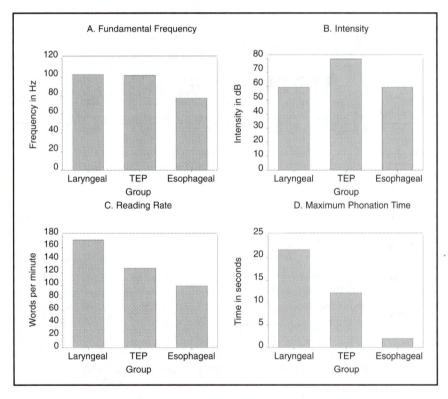

Figure 7–1. Some acoustic characteristics of alaryngeal speech. Laryngeal refers to a group of normal speakers, TE to a group of tracheoeophageal speakers and esoph to a group of esophageal speakers. (Drawn from data presented by Robbins, J. A., Fisher, H. B., Blom, E. D., & Singer, M. I. [1984]. A comparative acoustic study of normal, esophageal, and tracheo-esophageal speech production. *Journal of Speech and Hearing Disorders, 492,* 202–210.)

2. The F_0 of the **esophageal voice** is typically about 1 octave lower than the average laryngeal F_0 of a male voice, whereas the female esophageal voice is about 2 octaves lower than normal. Some of these data are shown in Table 7–1. Better esophageal speakers tend to produce somewhat higher F_0s whereas poorer speakers may produce somewhat lower F_0s. In a study by Slavin and Ferrand (1995), 26 esophageal speakers were clearly grouped according to their average F_0 and variability characteristics even though they were all proficient and highly intelligible speakers. Many esophageal speakers have difficulty controlling their F_0 during dynamic speech. Consequently, esophageal speakers exhibit greater variability than normal speakers. Some authors believe the F_0 of esophageal voice depends on the exact location of the vibrating segment, but there is little evidence to support this hypothesis.

Table 7–1. Fundamental frequency characteristics of alaryngeal speech. All data are reported from an oral reading of a reasonably long paragraph.

Study	N	Sex	Mean (Hz)	SD (ST)	Range (ST)
Esophageal Speech					
Damste, 1958	20		67.50[a]		
Snidecor & Curry, 1959	6	M	62.80	4.80	
Shipp, 1967	16[b]	M	64.74	4.98	16.00
	17[c]	M	84.40	4.54	15.20
Weinberg & Bennett, 1972	15	F	86.65	3.94	21.25
	18	M	57.40	4.15	23.76
Robbins et al., 1984	15	M	77.10	4.43	34.23
Tracheoesophageal Speech					
Robbins et al., 1984	15	M	101.70	3.56	37.46
Trudeau & Qi, 1990	10	F	108.6	2.68	
Moon & Weinberg, 1987	5	M	72.73[d]	0.91	22.44
Merwin et al., 1985	8	M	83.80[e]		
			78.70[f]		

[a]Median
[b]Rated below a 3 on a 7-point acceptability scale where 0 is least acceptable.
[c]Rated above a 3 on a 7-point acceptability scale where 0 is least acceptable.
[d]Phonation produced at comfortable effort level.
[e]Vowel /a/
[f]Vowel /i

3. **Tracheoesophageal speakers** tend to produce F_0s that are closer to normal laryngeal speakers, at least for male speakers. The variability of F_0 is also somewhat less than esophageal speakers, but individual speakers may show considerable variation.

B.   Vocal Intensity

1. Users of an **electrolarynx** can produce average intensity levels (see Figure 7–1B) during speech ranging between 75 and 85 dB, depending on the type of speech material (see Table 7–2). This level is typical of normal laryngeal speakers during ordinary conversation or reading. There is some evidence for a reduced intensity range for users of electrolarynges. As was the case for F_0, the intensity of the electronic vibrator is largely determined by the design of the instrument.

Table 7–2 Intensity characteristics of alaryngeal speech. All data reported in dB except where noted.

Study	N	Sex	Mean	SD	Range
Electrolarynx					
Hyman, 1955	8	M	83.00[a]		7.00
Weiss & Yeni-Komshian, 1979	5	M[e]	74.00	1.87	5.00
Esophageal Speech					
Hyman, 1955	7	M	73.00[a]	11.00	
Snidecor & Isshiki, 1965	1	M	85.00[b]	20.00	
Hoops and Noll, 1969	22	M	62.40[a]	3.60	10.55
Baggs & Pine, 1983	5	M	8.96[c]	1.58	4.33[c]
Robbins et al., 1984	15	M	59.30[a]		10.09[d]
				73.80[b]	3.50
Tracheoesophageal Speech					
Robbins et al., 1984	15	M	79.40[a]	2.10	13.8[d]
				88.10[b]	1.20
Baggs & Pine, 1983	5	M	19.56[c]	3.22[c]	15.69[c]
Trudeau & Qi, 1990	10	F	70.80[a]	8.50	29.00

[a]Reading passage.
[b]Sustained vowel.
[c]Reported in mm from a graphic level recording. Not converted to dB.
[d]Interquartile range.
[e]Subjects were normal speakers using an electrolarynx.

2. The intensity of **esophageal speech** is more variable and somewhat lower in overall loudness than normal. The range of voice intensity that esophageal speakers are able to produce is much less than the intensity range of normal laryngeal speakers (about 10 dB vs. 30 dB).

3. The intensity of **tracheoesophageal speech** appears to be only slightly less than the levels produced by laryngeal speakers. Variation of intensity may be somewhat greater than normal speakers. Some tracheoesophageal speakers habitually produce greater than normal intensity levels.

C. Perturbation

1. **Frequency perturbation (jitter)** reflects the frequency stability of the vocal folds. There are several measures developed to reflect jitter including mean period difference, jitter ratio, jitter factor, relative average perturbation (RAP), and directional perturbation. Jitter ratio and directional jitter have been used to measure frequency perturbation in alaryngeal speech. Jitter ratio is the ratio of the average period difference and the average period. Directional jitter is the number of sign changes of the period differences divided by the total number of periods. This ratio is then multiplied by 100 to yield a percentage measurement. Some data from the literature are reported in Table 7–3.

   a. There are no reported studies of frequency perturbation in speakers using an **electrolarynx**. However, jitter would be expected to be directly related to the stability of the electronic circuit producing the tone and would not reflect the speech characteristics of the speaker.

   b. **Esophageal** speech is more unstable than normal laryngeal speech as reflected in much larger jitter ratios. However, directional jitter is about the same magnitude as normal speakers. The tendency for esophageal speakers to oscillate up and down from an average frequency is about the same as normal speakers but the degree of their oscillatory differences is much greater than normal.

   c. The data on jitter characteristics of **tracheoesophageal** speakers are unclear. One study reports a jitter ratio very similar to normal speakers, whereas another reports a much

Table 7–3 Perturbation characteristics of alaryngeal speech.

Measure	Mean	SD	Range
Esophageal Speech[1]			
Jitter ratio	182.50	97.50	
Directional jitter(%)	58.70	13.40	
Shimmer (dB)	1.90	0.70	
Directional shimmer(%)	53.90	7.80	
Tracheoesophageal Speech			
Jitter ratio	51.40[1]	46.80[1]	
	134.80[2]	74.90[2]	255.40[2]
Directional jitter(%)	63.40[1]	9.30[1]	
	63.20[2]	7.70[2]	23.40[2]
Shimmer (dB)	0.80[1]	0.50[1]	
	1.90[2]	1.20[2]	3.90[2]
Directional shimmer(%)	62.90[1]	9.00[1]	
	64.90[2]	5.30[2]	17.40[2]
Normal[1]			
Jitter ratio	7.70	5.10	
Directional jitter(%)	54.30	8.60	
Shimmer (dB)	0.30	0.10	
Directional shimmer(%)	52.50	6.10	

[1]Robbins et al., 1984. Fifteen male esophageal, 15 male tracheoesophageal and 15 normal speakers produced the vowel /a/. A 1-second segment was used for the analysis of jitter and shimmer.
[2]Trudeau and Qi, 1990. Nine female tracheoesophageal speakers prolonged the vowel /a/.

higher than normal value. It would be reasonable to expect jitter values to be similar to (or perhaps even greater than) those of esophageal speakers as both groups of speakers use the same anatomical system as the vibrator, that is, the PE segment.

2. **Amplitude perturbation (shimmer)**, another index of the stability of a sound source, is a measure of the amplitude of vibration. It is typically expressed as the average difference in amplitude between adjacent cycles of vibration and is reported in dB. Directional shimmer, like directional jitter, is the number of changes of sign between adjacent periods divided by the total number of period differences, again multiplied by 100.

a. Shimmer in speakers using an **electrolarynx** would be expected to reflect the electronic design and construction of the instrument and not the inherent anatomical or physiological capabilities of the speaker.

b. Shimmer of **esophageal** speakers is greater than normal whereas directional shimmer is very similar to normal speakers.

c. Although the data are meager, it appears that both shimmer and directional shimmer are greater in **tracheoesophageal** than in normal speakers.

D. Temporal Characteristics

There have been a variety of temporal measurements (see Figure 7–1C and 7–1D) reported on alaryngeal speech, including words per minute (wpm), syllables per second, total duration of reading, words or syllables per air charge, and maximum duration of phonation. Table 7–4 shows three of these measurements chosen primarily because they appeared in many of the studies cited and because they appear to have some relevance to the acceptability and intelligibility of alaryngeal speech. The first is wpm as a measure of speech rate. The second is percentage of silence during reading

Table 7–4. Temporal characteristics of alaryngeal speech.

Type of Speaker	Sex	Mean	SD	Range
Words per Minute				
Esophageal	M[1]	113.00		
	M[2]	*		80–153
	M[3]	114.30		65.4–169
	M[4]	100.10	23.4	35.9–129.4
	M[5]	99.10	24.80	
Tracheoesophageal	M[5]	127.50	21.10	
	F[6]	138.03	39.70	87.5–198.6
Normal	M[5]	172.80	23.30	
Percent Silence				
Esophageal	M[7]	45.80		
		38.60		
	M[7]	29.61		
	F[8]	29.86		
	M[9]	34.79	7.24	29–47.26
	M[5]	33.40	11.30	
Tracheoesophageal	M[9]	18.70	8.96	4.92–29.23
	M[5]	10.50	10.40	
	F[6]	31.10	12.20	17–52
Normals	M[5]	11.60	6.0	

(continued)

Table 7–4. *(continued)*

Type of Speaker	Sex	Mean	SD	Range
Total Vowel Duration‡				
Esophageal	M[2]			0.39–0.51
	M[8]	5.49		
	F[8]	5.44		
	M[9]	4.82	1.70	2.47–7.10
	M[5]	1.90	0.70	
Tracheoesophageal	M[9]	11.00	4.58	6.97–17.60
	M[5]	12.20	5.20	
Normal	M[5]	21.80	9.10	

[1]Snidecor & Curry, 1959. Six superior male esophageal speakers read the Rainbow Passage.

[2]Snidecor & Isshiki, 1965. Six superior male esophageal speakers read a simple propositional paragraph and the Rainbow Passage.

[3]Hoops & Noll, 1969. Twenty-two male esophageal speakers read the Rainbow Passage.

[4]Filter & Hyman, 1975. Ten male and 10 female good esophageal speakers read a prose selection, a list of words from an intelligibility test, and a list of nonsense syllables.

[5]Robbins, Fisher, Blom, & Singer, 1984. Fifteen male laryngeal, 15 male esophageal and 15 male tracheoesophageal speakers prolonged the vowel /a/ for a long as possible and read the first paragraph of the Rainbow Passage.

[6]Trudeau & Qi, 1990. Ten female tracheoesophageal speakers read the Rainbow Passage and produced maximum duration on the vowel /a/.

[7]Shipp, 1967. Thirty-three male esophageal speakers read the Rainbow Passage. Second sentence was analyzed. One hundred sixty-six students rated each sentence on a 7-point speech acceptability scale where 1 was least acceptable and 5 most acceptable. Two groups were created, 16 whose average acceptability rating was below 3 and 17 with an average acceptability rating greater than 3.

[8]Weinberg &Bennett, 1972. Fifteen female and 18 male esophageal speakers read the Rainbow Passage.

[9]Baggs & Pine, 1983. Four male esophageal, 5 male tracheoesophageal, and 5 male laryngeal speakers read 14 sentences and prolonged the vowels /a/, /i/, and /u/ for as long as they could.

*No mean data reported.

‡This measure is referred to by a variety of names in the literature including maximum phonation duration or maximum vowel duration.

aloud, used here as a measure of pause time. The third is total vowel duration, or the maximum time a speaker can sustain a vowel. To a large extent, all of these measures reflect the speaker's ability to control the egressive air stream. For the esophageal speaker, they also reflect the ability to quickly recharge the esophagus with sufficient air. On many of these measures, an esophageal speaker will be at a disadvantage because of the small air volumes present in the esophagus, whereas tracheoesophageal speakers have the full pulmonary air supply. For users of an electrolarynx, phonation time is dependent on the vibrator, and silence is dependent on the speaker's facility with the on/off button.

1. The reading rate of **normal adults speakers** (between 40 and 70 years of age; ages most appropriate for comparison with laryngectomies) is about 173 wpm. Rates much less than 140 wpm are usually perceived as slow and rates above 185 wpm are perceived as fast (Franke, 1939). Normal speakers can produce about 13 words per breath of air, which averages to about 4 seconds in duration (Snidecor & Curry, 1959).

2. There are few data on the **temporal characteristics of speech produced with an electrolarynx.** The few studies available tend to indicate that reading rates are slower when using an electrolarynx compared to normal phonation or to tracheoesophageal speech (Merwin et al., 1985; Weiss & Yeni-Komshian, 1979). We might expect longer reading times for electrolarynx users because of the need to produce more precise articulation to maintain an acceptable level of intelligibility.

3. In general, **esophageal** speakers read slower than normal laryngeal speakers. Rates between 100–115 wpm appear typical for these speakers, which is about 60–70% of the rate of normal speakers. Esophageal speakers generally spend about 30–45% of their reading time in silence. These abnormally long silent periods reflect the more frequent need to recharge air supply. Better esophageal speakers have much shorter periods of silence indicating more rapid air intake with less interruption of speech flow. Esophageal speakers also have a much shorter sustained duration of "phonation" than normal speakers, typically less than 6 seconds (vs. 15–20 seconds for normal speakers). This no doubt reflects the small volume of air in the esophagus.

4. **Tracheoesophageal speakers** also read at a slower rate than normal speakers but faster than esophageal speakers. Their slower rate may reflect difficulty in controlling the PE segment and the need to articulate precisely. These speakers spend about 10–30% of their time in silence, shorter than esophageal speakers and comparable to or slightly longer than normal speakers. This is probably reflective of the ability to use full pulmonary air supply to drive the PE segment. Tracheoesophageal speakers also can produce long phonation durations (about 12 seconds) for the same reason.

II. PHYSIOLOGICAL CHARACTERISTICS

A. Mechanisms of Air Intake

1. The classic study of Diedrich and Youngstrom (1966) demonstrated that esophageal speakers used two mechanisms (injection and inhalation) to obtain air for phonation.

2. **Injection** refers to the process in which air in the oral cavity is pushed back into the pharynx and esophagus by action of the tongue. The velopharyngeal sphincter must close to prevent escape of air through the nose. Highly tonic PE segments may prevent air from entering the esophagus.

3. **Inhalation** takes advantage of the lower than normal pressure within the esophagus by relaxing the PE segment and allowing air to move from the region of high pressure in the mouth or from outside the mouth into the slightly negative region in the esophagus, in a manner similar to normal respiratory function.

B. Mechanisms of Vibration

1. Little is known about the **vibratory characteristics** of the PE segment. Many believe that it is controlled by both an aerodynamic and a myoelastic process in much the same manner as laryngeal phonation. For example, there appears to be a mucosal wave, a ripple-like motion of the esophagus appearing beneath the neoglottis and moving upward. A mucosal wave is an important feature of normal vocal fold motion.

2. Moon and Weinberg (1987) have demonstrated that pitch control in TEP speakers (and probably to some degree in esophageal speakers) is primarily **aerodynamically controlled**, but in some cases myoelastic factors may be operating. In most cases, they found that pitch raised or lowered with increases or decreases of airflow, although some subjects could vary pitch without systemically altering airflow rate. This suggests that there is some measure of muscle control of the PE segment and that speakers can learn to control these muscles sufficiently for pitch control during speech. If so, speakers with this control should produce better and more intelligible speech. However, even TEP speakers exhibited considerable variability in their pitch control, airflow, and tracheal pressures.

3. Omori, Kojiman, Nonomura, and Fukushima (1994) have recently elucidated the possible mechanism of vibration in tracheoesophageal speakers by studying the vibration of the shunt in 25 tracheoesophageal speakers (all but one male) using stroboscopy, fluoroscopy, and EMG. From their fluoroscopy studies, they reported two bulges in the neck, the first typically located between C-4 and C-6 and the second typically located at about C-5 to C-7. Stroboscopy demonstrated that the upper bulge was vibrating during phonation in all patients. No vibration was observed in the lower bulge. From their EMG studies, they concluded that the muscle comprising the upper bulge is the thyropharyngeus muscles whereas the lower bulge is composed of the cricopharyngeus muscle. It would appear from this study that the muscle controlling vibration in tracheoesophageal speakers is the thyropharyngeus and not the cricopharyngeus that has been reported in the past to control the vibrating PE sphincter in esophageal speakers and thought to be responsible for vibration in tracheoesophageal speakers.

C. Articulatory Characteristics

1. Considerable **tongue** activity is necessary for esophageal speakers who use the injection method for air intake. The tongue is also necessary for producing individual speech sounds. The need of esophageal speakers to place the tongue in certain postures prior to producing speech to inject or inhale air may affect the position of the tongue during the production of the speech sound. For example, during air intake, the tongue is close to the hard palate. To produce vowels requiring a low tongue position, the tongue must move a greater distance when a speaker uses the injection method than in any other method of speech. Thus, the tendency of a person using the injection method to produce esophageal speech would be to produce all low vowels with a higher than usual tongue position, a tendency confirmed by evidence (Hoops & Noll, 1969).

2. Formant frequencies may be higher in esophageal (and perhaps TEP) speakers, suggesting a shorter vocal tract (Christensen & Weinberg, 1976). Speakers may be able to compensate for the shorter vocal tract by pursing their lips more or altering their tongue position.

3. Vowel durations in the connected speech of esophageal speakers are longer than normal suggesting changed articulatory dynamics as well as the slower rate of speaking. Longer vowel durations may also reflect the inability of esophageal and TE speakers to start and stop voicing, as compared to laryngeal speakers. This voicing control problem is also reflected in the inability of esophageal and TEP speakers to produce the voiced/voiceless distinction consistently.

III. PERCEPTUAL CHARACTERISTICS

A. Intelligibility

1. The intelligibility of speech (see Figure 7–2) can be **assessed** in a variety of ways. A trained listener could analyze and precisely transcribe the speech produced. This is sometimes referred to as an articulation score. Or, a listener might be instructed to write down the word spoken or choose a response from a list of four to six alternatives. On a more general level, a listener could

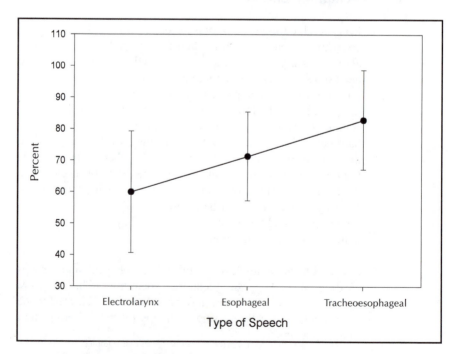

Figure 7–2. Intelligibility of alaryngeal speech. These data are drawn from various sources and are composite data.

simply judge the intelligibility of speech by rating it on a 5- or 7-point scale. All of these methods have been used to describe the intelligibility of alaryngeal speech. Different assessment methods yield different results. The results shown in Table 7–5

Table 7–5. Intelligibility of alaryngeal speech.

Study	Percent
Electrolarynx Speech	
Hyman, 1955[1]	43.60
McCroskey & Milligan, 1963[2]	60.30
Weiss & Yeni-Komshian, 1979[3]	89.60
Kalb & Carpenter, 1981	70.73[4]
	61.81[5]
Weiss & Basili, 1985	32.50[6]
	36.33[7]
Merwin et al., 1985[8]	65.55
Blom, Singer, & Hamaker, 1986[9]	79.55
Average (Standard Deviation)	60.00 (19.34)
Esophageal Speech	
Hyman, 1955[1]	49.20
McCroskey & Mulligan,1963[2]	58.20
Hoops & Curtis, 1971[10]	75.13
Horii & Weinberg, 1975[11]	95-98
Filter & Hyman, 1975[12]	78.15
Swisher, 1980[13]	66.20
Kalb & Carpenter, 1981	67.33[4]
	78.55[5]
Merwin et al.,1985[8]	70.80
Blom, Singer, & Hamaker,1986[9]	88.74
Doyle, Danhauer, & Reed, 1988[14]	55.90
Miralles & Cervera, 1995[16]	81.98
Average (Standard Deviation)	72.22 (14.23)
Tracheoesophageal Speech	
Tardy-Mitzell et al., 1985[15]	93.00
Blom, Singer, & Hamaker, 1986[9]	91.00
Doyle, Danhauer, & Reed, 1988[14]	64.80
Miralles & Cervera,1995[16]	84.48
Average (Standard Deviation)	83.32 (12.87)

[1] Eight good esophageal speakers or eight electrolarynx speakers read the Black Multiple Choice Intelligibility Test. Twelve listeners were used.

[2] Five esophageal and five electrolarynx speakers read a multiple choice intelligibility test. Ten naive listeners made their choice from four alternatives.

(continued)

Table 7–5. *(continued)*

[3]Five normal speaking male adults read the modified rhyme word lists using a Western Electric model 5 electrolarynx. Eight female listeners chose their response from among six alternatives.

[4]Five esophageal speakers who also used an electrolarynx read the Harvard PB word lists. Thirty naive listeners wrote down what they heard.

[5]Five speakers who used only esophageal speech and five speakers who used only a electro-larynx read the Harvard PB word lists. Thirty naive listeners wrote down what they heard.

[6]Six males using the Western Electric model 5 electrolarynx read a 66-word list consisting of CVC syllables. Six speech-language pathology students transcribed the lists.

[7]Six males using the Servox electrolarynx read a 66-word list consisting of CVC syllables. Six speech-language pathology students transcribed the lists.

[8]Eight male speakers, seven of whom used an electrolarynx and one who was an esophageal speaker read the Black Multiple Choice Intelligibility test. All later received a tracheoesophageal puncture and read the lists again. Forty-five speech pathology majors served as listeners.

[9]Twenty-seven electrolarynx and seven esophageal speakers spoke the Modified Rhyme Test. Eighty naive listeners chose from one of six alternatives.

[10]Twenty-eight esophageal speakers, rated from poor to superior in proficiency, read sentence lists and the Rainbow Passage. Twenty-one experienced speech-language pathologists supplied the words to complete the sentence.

[11]Two superior male esophageal speakers read lists of the Consonant and Vowel Rhyme tests. Sixteen college students chose their response from among six alternatives.

[12]Twenty esophageal speakers (10 male and 10 female) read the Black Multiple Choice Intelligibility Tests. Ten speech-language pathology students transcribed the lists.

[13]Ten male esophageal speakers read CVC syllables in a carrier phrase. Twenty-five speech-language pathology students wrote down the syllable heard.

[14]Three esophageal, three tracheoesophageal and one subject who used both forms of communication spoke a CVCVC utterance in a carrier phrase with the V being either /i/ or /u/ and the C one of the 24 English consonants. Fifteen naive listeners wrote down what they heard.

[15]Five female and 10 male tracheoesophageal speakers read the House consonant word lists. Forty-six naive listeners made judgments of the intelligibility of the speaker using a 7-point scale.

[16]Twenty tracheoesophageal and 10 male esophageal Spanish speaker read a list of 24 Spanish two-syllable words. One hundred forty listeners listened to the tape-recorded samples and wrote down the word they heard.

have been obtained using reasonably comparable methods, although some of the variation among the results may be due partly to procedural differences among the studies cited.

2. Generally, the most **proficient** speakers have been used as subjects as the intent was to determine how intelligible the different forms of alaryngeal speech can be. Thus, these data represent optimum results. However, these are targets that can be used for individual patients as they learn and master their chosen form of alaryngeal speech.

3. Few studies have compared all three forms of alaryngeal speech. Those that have show that tracheoesophageal speakers generally produce the highest intelligibility scores. Variability is the rule rather than the exception. Some excellent esophageal speakers can produce extremely intelligible speech, whereas poor or even some good tracheoesophageal speakers are much less intelligible. Speakers who have mastered an electrolarynx can produce speech that is much more intelligible than a mediocre esophageal or tracheoesophageal speaker.

4. The intelligibility of speakers using an **electrolarynx** ranges between 30 and 90%. The average intelligibility in the studies reported in Table 7–5 is 60%. The major detriment to intelligibility of this form of alaryngeal speech is the failure to maintain the voicing distinction. Voiceless consonants tend to sound like voiced consonants. It is very difficult for these speakers to start and stop the electronic vibrator to signal the presence of a voiceless consonant. In fact, most speakers do not attempt to do so. Rather, they learn to produce other cues (e.g., vowel duration before or after the consonant) that help to signal the voicing distinction. Fricative consonant production is also difficult for similar reasons. Alaryngeal speakers have difficulty producing the air pressures required to produce long duration and/or intense noise associated with these consonants. Increasing the intelligibility of stops and fricatives is a major task for the speech-language pathologist and the patient.

5. The intelligibility of **esophageal speech** varies considerably, but in general is somewhat higher than intelligibility for users of an electrolarynx. The average is about 72%. Some of this difference between electronic and esophageal speech may be due to speaker differences. One study (Kalb & Carpenter, 1981) found that there was little difference in intelligibility between proficient esophageal and proficient electrolarynx speakers.

a. Most of the **errors** exhibited by esophageal speakers were voicing errors. Like users of an electrolarynx, voiceless consonants were perceived as voiced. Fricatives and nasals were also difficult to understand in this form of alaryngeal speech.

b. In general, it appears that users of an electrolarynx and esophageal speakers exhibit many of the same kind of errors, probably for the same reasons. **Improving the articulation of alaryngeal speakers** appears to help their intelligibility.

6. **Tracheoesophageal speakers** also show considerable variation in intelligibility, but in general, they produce the most intelligible speech of the three forms of alaryngeal speech. This may be somewhat misleading as there are only four studies reported (see Table 7–5). It is also somewhat surprising because tracheoesophageal speakers use the same vibrator as esophageal speakers and may have very similar vocal tract and neck changes as speakers using either an electrolarynx or esophageal speech. However, tracheoesophageal speakers, because of their normal air supply, do not have to use any structures in the vocal tract to insufflate the PE segment, therefore they can maintain their normal (or develop normal) patterns of articulation and more normal flow of speech.

Tracheoesophageal speakers produce **errors** very similar to users of an electrolarynx or esophageal speech. Voicing is the major intelligibility error followed by production of fricatives and affricates. One would expect that tracheoesophageal speakers would have good ability to produce high pressures needed to produce long or intense noise sources needed for fricative or affricate production. Thus, the finding that they produce errors involving fricatives and affricates is somewhat puzzling. However, tracheoesophageal speakers may also need considerable air pressure simply to force air through the prosthesis into the esophagus and pharynx. The air pressures in the vocal tract may be reduced considerably by the time air reaches the pharynx. The need for higher than normal tracheal pressures has led to the development of low resistance prostheses.

a. One study (Williams, Scanlon, & Ritterman, 1989) examined temporal and perceptual characteristics of the speech of users of a regular and a low resistance prosthesis. Their judges rated intelligibility on a 7-point scale. However, no data were presented on the comparable intelligibility of the two devices.

b. In a study of Spanish-speaking esophageal and tracheo-esophageal speakers, Miralles and Cervera (1995) reported on an intelligibility study using 30 male speakers, most of whom had either a medium, or low pressure prosthesis. These authors did not specifically address any differences between high, medium, and low resistance prostheses but their results suggest that overall intelligibility is good in low pressure devices. They also analyzed the consonant confusions that were produced and found that the tracheoesophageal group produced a slightly greater percentage of correct responses for stops, glides, and nasals than did the esophageal group but the latter had a larger percentage of correct responses for the fricatives. The results are illustrated in Figure 7–3.

7. To a large extent, the intelligibility of alaryngeal speech depends on the **unique characteristics** of the speaker rather than the unique characteristics of the form of alaryngeal speech. There are anatomical changes that have been made in the speaker's vocal tract and perhaps the esophagus that may affect that speaker's ability to speak again or to speak well with the new form of speech. The individual skill of the speaker in learning the various compensatory strategies needed to produce intelligible speech is another important factor that affects outcome.

a. **The form of alaryngeal speech may not limit intelligibility.** A good speaker with an electrolarynx may be better than an average speaker using esophageal speech. In one study, persons were equally intelligible with an electrolarynx and esophageal speech (Kalb & Carpenter, 1981). Drummond, Dancer, Krueger, and Spring, (1996) found that in their group of eight male alaryngeal speakers using either an artifical device or tracheoesophageal speech the most important factors for assessing alaryngeal connected speech were vocal quality, understandability, extraneous speaking noise, and overall communication effectiveness.

b. **Intelligibility should be assessed** under a variety of conditions and with different types of material. Individual words are seldom used in everyday conversation, however, tests using individual words may be good predictors of conversational intelligibility. Sentences and paragraphs are probably the best stimuli to use for estimating intelligibility. Patients

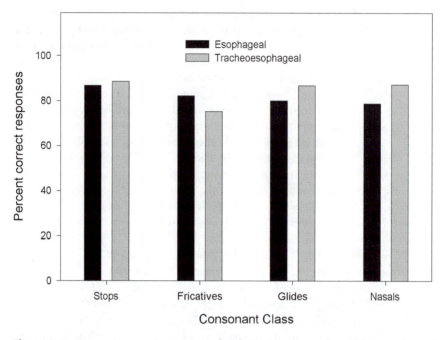

Figure 7–3. Percent correct responses for four consonant classes for esophageal and tracheoesophageal speakers of Spanish. (Data drawn from Miralles, J. L., & Cervera, T. [1995]. Voice intelligibility in patients who have undergone laryngectomies. *Journal of Speech and Hearing Research, 38*[3], 564–571.)

should be taught and encouraged to monitor their intelligibility and develop practice patterns to improve it. Self-administered intelligibility tests may be excellent tools to improve the intelligibility of alaryngeal speakers (Fitzpatrick, Gould, & Nichols, 1980).

c. In all forms of alaryngeal speech, it is necessary for speakers to develop **compensatory cues** to mark voicing, and in some instances, manner of production as well. All modes of alaryngeal speech indicate difficulty producing the noise or noise bursts needed to signal a voiceless consonant, especially voiceless stops. However, presence or absence of noise is not the only cue for voicing. The duration, F_0, and intensity levels of the preceding or following vowel are also different. Speakers can use some of these features to signal the voiced or voiceless consonant.

d. It is clear from the literature that **tracheoesophageal speech is very intelligible** although not as intelligible as normal laryngeal speech. This may be due to the presence of a large air supply that can be controlled independently from the vocal tract, permitting the production of long uninterrupted speech units. It may also assist the speaker in maintaining normal flow and rate of speaking because of the greater volume of air and the absence of frequent interruptions needed to ingress air as in esophageal speech. But both tracheoesophageal and esophageal speakers use the same vibrator and some of their speech characteristics are dependent on the capabilities and limitations of the vibrator formed by the PE segment.

e. The **types of errors** produced by all forms of alaryngeal speech are very similar although they differ in degree. Thus, some of the same therapeutic strategies can be used with all forms of alaryngeal speech.

f. Finally, it is wise to remember that **intelligibility may depend partly on the listener**—what the listener expects to hear, the listener's familiarity with alaryngeal speech and/or the listener's own experience with laryngectomized persons. Naive listeners provide lower intelligibility scores than expert listeners. Expert listeners may place more importance on certain useful perceptual or acoustic characteristics than do either laryngectomized persons or naive listeners. The patient and clinician should know the intended or expected audience when evaluating a patient's intelligibility.

B.   Acceptability/Preference

1. **Acceptability** of alaryngeal speech certainly does not mean that a listener prefers that voice. A preferred voice must be acceptable but an acceptable voice may not be preferred. However, the ranking of voices along an acceptability scale may provide some insight into the preferences of the listener.

2. In general, **excellent TE speakers are preferred** over excellent esophageal speakers. Excellent speakers with an electrolarynx may be as good as either tracheoesophageal or esophageal speakers. In some cases, a good electrolarynx user or a user of a pneumatic speech aid may be preferred to a poor esophageal speaker. All forms of alaryngeal speech may be acceptable to listeners if the speaker is reasonably proficient in that form of speech.

3. **Excellent female esophageal or tracheoesophageal speakers** may be more acceptable (or even preferred) to excellent male speakers in either category. There is little difference in acceptability between good and excellent male speakers.

4. The **acceptability of alaryngeal speech** does not appear to depend on the age of the speaker. Older, but proficient, speakers using any form of alaryngeal speech are preferred to younger, less proficient speakers.

5. Among esophageal and tracheoesophageal speakers there is little difference between those judged good and those judged excellent. The proficiency of the speaker has more to do with acceptability of alaryngeal speech than the specific form of speech used. Of course, in general, it may be more difficult for esophageal speakers to become proficient than it is for tracheoesophageal speakers.

6. Patients who use tracheoesophageal speech are generally more satisfied with the quality of their speech and with their ability to communicate over the telephone. Furthermore, they feel less limited in their interactions with others (Clements et al., 1997).

IV. PERCEPTUAL CHARACTERISTICS (SEE FIGURE 7–4)

A. Pitch

1. All alaryngeal speakers are usually perceived to possess an abnormal pitch level. Potentially, the **pitch of electrolarynx** users may be least affected as the appropriate pitch level can be set within the instrument.

2. **Esophageal speakers** are generally perceived to have a **very low pitch** which correlates with the low F_0 they produce. In some instances, a male speaker may produce a pitch that is perceived only slightly lower than a normal male voice.

3. **Tracheoesophageal speakers** may also exhibit a low pitch level although not as low as esophageal speakers. Through practice, it is possible to develop a pitch more appropriate to normal male

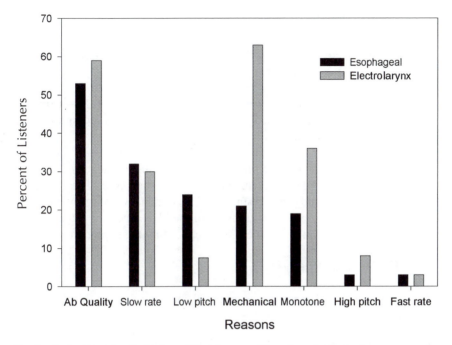

Figure 7–4. Perceived abnormalities in esophageal and electrolarynx speech. (Drawn from data presented by Bennett, S., & Weinberg, B. [1973]. Acceptability ratings of normal, esophageal, and artificial larynx speech. *Journal of Speech and Hearing Research, 16,* 608–615.)

voices, although female tracheoesophageal speakers may continue to have a lower than normal pitch level.

4. In all forms of alaryngeal speech, some speakers may develop a higher than expected or desired pitch level.

B. Loudness

1. **Esophageal speakers** tend to produce **lower than normal loudness** levels. This can make it somewhat difficult to hear esophageal speech, particularly in the presence of high ambient noise levels. Sometimes, the low loudness levels may be masked by stoma blast (the sound produced when excessive force is used in pushing air through the stoma).

2. **Electrolarynx and tracheoesophageal speakers** are usually capable of producing normal or near normal loudness levels.

C. Quality

1. Almost all laryngeal speakers are perceived to have **an abnormal voice quality**.

2. Listeners usually perceive speech produced with an **electrolarynx** as mechanical or robot-like. They may complain of a monotone quality.

3. Listeners often think that esophageal or tracheoesophageal speakers have severe laryngitis or a bad cold. The quality is hoarse and rough sounding. The combination of a low pitch and the vibratory characteristics of the PE segment produce a sound that is similar to vocal fry produced by the normal larynx.

D. Rate of Speaking

1. **Electrolarynx and esophageal speakers** are perceived to have a slow rate of speaking.

2. **Tracheoesophageal speakers** are perceived to speak at normal or near normal rates.

3. **A slow rate of speech** may interfere with intelligibility, thereby interfering with the speaker's ability to communicate.

E. Other Factors

1. Many alaryngeal speakers are perceived to speak in a **monotone**. In the case of electrolarynx users, the perception may result from the lack of variability in the sound source. In the case of esophageal or tracheoesophageal speech, the problem may reflect an inability to vary pitch voluntarily while speaking. In addition, because it is difficult to start and stop vibration of the PE segment, the tendency to continue voicing through the aperiodic or silent portions of speech may contribute to the perception of a monotone.

2. **Electrolarynx users** will have a "voice" quality determined by the instrument used. Most sound sources are pulse-like, producing greater energy in the higher harmonics. Pulse waveforms sound harsher and are perceived to be more unpleasant than other waveforms.

F. Influence of Abnormal Acoustic Factors

1. Alaryngeal speakers exhibit a variety of **abnormal acoustic factors**. However, not all of these factors may contribute equally to the acceptability or the intelligibility of the speech.

   a. For example, **rate and loudness** appear to be important in the acceptability of electrolarynx speech but are less important for the other two forms of alaryngeal speech (Williams & Williams, 1989).

   b. **Pitch and quality** appear to be important in the acceptability of esophageal speech.

   c. **Pitch, quality, and loudness** are important determinants of the acceptability of tracheoesophageal speech.

2. The **experience of the listener** can also determine the degree to which abnormal speech factors affect the acceptability of alaryngeal speech (Watson & Williams, 1987).

   a. **Laryngectomees** rate the three forms of alaryngeal speech differently than naive or expert listeners.

   b. Laryngectomees are not as critical about **pitch or rate** as they are about the visual appearance of the speaker while speaking.

   c. Laryngectomees are less critical about the **pitch and quality** of esophageal speech than are naive listeners.

   d. Rate of speaking is more important to laryngectomee listeners than to naive or expert listeners.

G. Effect of Tracheostoma Valves on Speech

There are a number of valves available that allow for greater ease in speaking by "automatically" shunting the exhaled air from the lungs to the prosthesis for producing voice. These valves permit "hands free" speech and should not affect the quality of the speech produced. But they apparently do have an effect. Leder (1994) reported significant differences in speech quality ratings among the four valves he studied: Montgomery, Passy-Muir, Kistner, and Olympic. The Passy-Muir valve was identified as having the best speech quality.

Furthermore, this valve exhibited the fewest mechanical problems. The rankings of the four valves are shown in Figure 7–5.

V. SUMMARY

Acoustically, mechanical speech aids have a constant F_0 and sufficient intensity for everyday speech purposes. Esophageal speakers tend to produce lower than normal F_0s, a somewhat lower and more variable intensity, and greater frequency and amplitude perturbation. The F_0s of tracheoesophageal speakers are similar to laryngeal speakers but produce slightly lower intensities. The stability of the sound source, as measured by frequency and amplitude perturbation, appears similar to that of esophageal speakers.

Temporally, speakers who use a mechanical speech aid speak more slowly than normal speakers. Esophageal speakers speak at about 70%

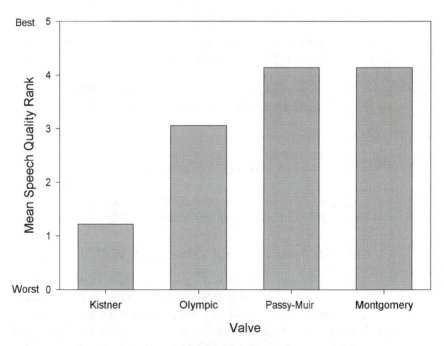

Figure 7–5. Ranking of speech intelligibility among four speaking valves. (Data drawn from Leder, S. B. [1994]. Perceptual rankings of speech quality produced with one-way tracheostomy speaking valves. *Journal of Speech and Hearing Research,* *37*[6], 1308–1312.)

of the rate of normal speakers but have a higher proportion of silent time. Tracheoesophageal speakers tend to speak slower than normal speakers but faster than esophageal speakers.

Esophageal and tracheoesophageal speakers use the same sound vibrator, that is, the PE segment. It is believed that vibration of the PE segment is controlled by aerodynamic and myoelastic factors. In most esophageal or tracheoesophageal speakers, unlike laryngeal speakers, F_0 appears to be controlled aerodynamically. Esophageal speakers use considerable tongue activity to move air into the esophagus. The active tongue may affect the articulation of some sounds. Their vowel durations are longer than normal.

The intelligibility of all forms of alaryngeal speech is generally lower than laryngeal speech. There is considerable variability among speakers, however. Some users of mechanical speech aids are very intelligible, whereas esophageal or even tracheoesophageal speakers can be much less intelligible. Most errors in all forms of alaryngeal speech are voicing errors. It is difficult to produce good voiceless consonants. Improving articulation helps to reduce these errors. In general, tracheoesophageal speech is preferred to esophageal or mechanically aided speech. Interestingly, an excellent female speaker may be preferred to an excellent male speaker. Older, but proficient, speakers are preferred to younger, less proficient speakers.

The pitch of all forms of alaryngeal speech is generally perceived to be abnormal; sometimes too low, other times too high. Tracheoesophageal speakers tend to show the least deviation from a laryngeal speaker. Esophageal speakers tend to produce softer speech than the other forms of alaryngeal speech and almost all alaryngeal speakers are perceived to have an abnormal "voice" quality. It is, however, somewhat difficult to predict which of the abnormal perceptual factors will affect a listener's acceptance of alaryngeal speech. Some listeners may be affected by the abnormal pitch, whereas others may dislike the quality. The experience of the listener also affects the weight given to the various abnormal perceptual factors.

In several areas, the results of research on the acoustic, physiologic, and perceptual aspects of alaryngeal speech are confusing and incomplete. Few studies have directly compared all forms of alaryngeal speech with sufficient subjects to draw meaningful conclusions. Results are often contradictory. This may be partially explained by the variability of alaryngeal speech. There are few data on the vibratory characteristics of the PE segment and its important control mechanisms. Manufacturers of speech aids have done little to build a better sound source except for occasional attempts to provide control of the F_0 of the tone. In this day of microchips and dynamic programming, it would seem possible to build a mechanical sound source that is more like the source produced by normal vocal folds, thus, reducing the mechanical sound. Advances in surgical techniques may someday produce a substitute vibrator that exhibits some of the important mechanical characteristics of normal vocal folds.

VI. SPEECH CHARACTERISTICS OF PATIENTS WITH GLOSSECTOMY

Although there are several articulators used during the production of speech, the tongue is the most important. It is active during the production of all vowels and most of the consonants. Variation of tongue position along the anteroposterior direction and in the cranial-caudal direction is very apparent during the production of vowels to produce the appropriate resonance changes. According to theory, variations along the anteroposterior direction affect the frequency of the second formant, an important acoustic cue to place of articulation. Variations in the cranial-caudal direction affect the degree of constriction in the vocal tract and affect F1 and F2 center frequencies. The tongue is essential for the production of many consonants, including /t/, /d/, /k/, /g/, /l/, /d /, /n/, and /r/. Consonants are very important to the overall intelligibility of speech. Removal of the tongue would be expected to reduce speech intelligibility severely. How severely intelligibility is reduced depends on the extent of tongue removal and the ability of the patient to manipulate the remaining portion. Patients who have had a glossectomy are expected to have severe problems communicating even if the larynx is spared (and in some cases it is not). In this section, a brief review of the speech characteristics of patients with partial or total glossectomy is presented.

A. Intelligibility of the Glossectomized

Several studies have reported on the intelligibility characteristics of patients with partial or total glossectomies. Unfortunately, many have reported on only one or two subjects, and there are meager data about the intelligibility of patients with glossectomy. The most extensive study reported on 14 total and 11 partial glossectomees (Skelly, Spector, Donaldsen, Brodeur, & Paletta, 1971). Six of the 14 total glossectomees also were dysphagic and an additional patient had a laryngectomy. All of these patients were virtually unintelligible. The intelligibility of the remaining total glossectomized and 7 of the partial glossectomees (3 left the therapy program) was assessed using the phonetically balanced (PB) word lists, lists of glossal monosyllables and a list of life situation questions. The results of the analysis prior to the start of a 12-month program of speech therapy are shown in Table 7–6. It is apparent that the total glossectomy group produced unintelligible speech across all conditions. They were even poor in communicating simple needs; a condition where context and situational factors would be expected to assist their ability to communicate. The partial glossectomy group produced intelligibility scores between 14 and 45%.

Other studies (usually with one patient) have reported similar intelligibility scores, although in one case of a total glossectomy (Leonard & Gillis, 1982) vowel intelligibility reached almost 50%. However, speech therapy and/or the use of a prosthesis can improve intelligibility scores for even the patient with a total glossectomy. In the study by Skelly et al. (1971), a program of therapy was designed that included exercises to improve flexibility of the available articulators, explored potential compensatory movements that could improve vowel and/or consonant intelligibility, and applied successful compensatory strategies learned by one patient to the other patients. Intelligibility was assessed at the end of 12 months, and the results are shown in Table 7–6 and Figure 7–6. Both groups had an increase in intelligibility. The total glossectomy group had the largest increase, especially for the life situation question task. Of course, they started with a lower score and had a greater potential for improvement. Partial glossectomy patients showed less of an increase especially for the glossal monosyllable word lists.

Table 7–6. Intelligibility in percent for partial and total glossectomees prior to a 12 month therapy program.

Type of Surgery	Words	Syllables	Questions
Partial	13.75	15.75	45.50
Total	5.71	0.86	4.00

Source: Data from Skelly, M., Donaldson, R. C., Fust, R. S., & Townsend, D. L. 1972. Changes in phonatory aspects of glossectomee intelligibility through vocal parameter manipulation. *Journal of Speech and Hearing Disorders, 37*, 379–389.

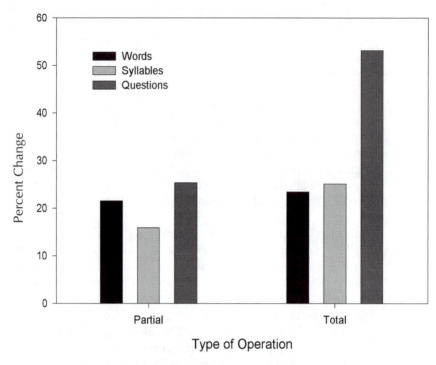

Figure 7–6. Change of intelligibility after a 12-month program of speech therapy for a group of partial and a group of total glossectomees. (Drawn from data presented by Skelly, M., Spector, D., Donaldson, R., Brodeur, A., & Paletta, F. [1971]. Compensatory physiologic phonetics for the glossectomee. *Journal of Speech and Hearing Disorders, 36,* 101–114.)

Speech therapy appears to be a viable alternative for patients with a partial glossectomy and with complete removal of the tongue who retain a viable residual mass. For most patients with a total glossectomy, the benefits of speech therapy are limited, but other options may be considered such as further reconstructive surgery or a prosthesis. In these cases, speech therapy can also be of benefit.

B. Acoustic Characteristics of the Speech of the Glossectomized

One would expect that sounds requiring tongue movement would be most affected by partial or total glossectomy. The available evidence supports this conclusion. Vowels requiring a high or frontal tongue position will be most affected. Several studies have reported little effect of glossectomy on the center frequency of the first formant, because its frequency is affected mostly by the lips and to some degree by jaw opening. The most pronounced effect is on the center frequency of the second formant (Georgian, Logemann, & Fisher, 1982; LaRiviere, Seilo, & Dimmick, 1975; Leonard & Gillis, 1983; Morrish, 1984; Skelly et al., 1972). The frequency of the second formant is affected by the amount and place of constriction within the oral cavity. For example, as a constriction in the oral cavity is moved from the soft palate to the alveolar ridge, the frequency of the second formant rises. The amount of frequency change is affected by the degree of constriction. To obtain the necessary constriction, the tongue must be raised toward the hard palate and moved from the teeth to the soft palate. Patients with reasonable amounts of tongue mass (e.g., 20–30% or more) may be able to achieve the appropriate constrictions. Patients with little tongue mass may have to develop compensatory movements to produce the appropriate acoustics. Some patients use the pharynx, epiglottis, any residual tongue mass (or in some cases flaps fashioned at the time of surgery), and jaw movement (lowering/elevation and/or protrusion/retraction).

Consonants requiring the use of the tongue would be misarticulated by patients with partial and total glossectomy. In one report (Georgian et al., 1982) of the consonant errors of one patient with 20% of the tongue removed and the remaining portion sutured to the floor of the mouth, the most common error was place misarticulation. The patient used jaw protrusion or retraction to compensate for the poor tongue mobility. Similar compensatory adjustments were noted for the production of consonants by two subjects with a total glossectomy (Morrish, 1984, 1988). One of these patients could not produce good velars because of the small residual tongue mass. In some patients, jaw lowering helped to differentiate high from low vowels.

Partial glossectomees should learn to use their residual tongue mass to its maximum potential. Even with 50% loss of tongue mass, vowel and consonant articulation may be very good. Total glossectomees can develop compensatory articulatory patterns that may improve their vowel and consonant intelligibility. However, one should expect deficiencies for consonants or vowels requiring high tongue position. Knowledge of the relationships between articulator movements and the resonant patterns produced can be very helpful in developing compensatory strategies and improving those a patient may have already learned.

C. Effects of a Tongue Prosthesis

In total glossectomy, a patient may have so little residual tongue mass or other limitations, that speech is unintelligible. It may be appropriate to consider an oral prosthesis that may restore some of the tongue function. Several reports have appeared (Leonard & Gillis, 1982, 1983, 1990) in which the effects of a tongue prosthesis on speech articulation have been reported. In one patient with total glossectomy, vowel intelligibility increased from 48% to 64% with a custom made prosthesis anchored to the mandibular teeth. Fewer place errors were noted, and the patient produced better examples of front and back vowels. Apparently, the prosthesis allowed the patient to achieve some degree of constriction along the anteroposterior dimension of the vocal tract. In a later study on the same patient (Leonard et al., 1983), the range of F2 center frequency increased with the prosthesis in place, no doubt contributing to the increased vowel intelligibility.

In a study of 5 patients with partial and total glossectomy (Leonard & Gillis, 1990), the effects of a prosthesis on vowel and consonant intelligibility was assessed. With the prostheses in place, intelligibility improved about 12%, the range of F2 center frequency widened by about 20%, and the number of consonant errors decreased by about 14% (see Table 7–7 and Figure 7–7). Interestingly, the patient with the most severe surgery (bilateral extensive removal) improved the most.

A prosthesis placed appropriately in the oral cavity, with consideration for swallowing, can improve the speech production abilities of patients with total or partial glossectomies. However, a prosthesis may affect a patient's speech production abilities in different ways, depending on the amount of residual mass, mobility of the tongue, extent of surgery, and other factors. A prosthesis must be fashioned according to the unique needs and capabilities of the patient. One should assess the exact errors produced with the prosthesis and alter the prosthesis to correct those specific errors.

Table 7–7. Intelligibility severity, F2 center frequency range, and number of error consonants with and without a prosthesis.

Severity Scale (1–7)		F2 Range (% Normal)		No Consonants in Error	
With	*Without*	*With*	*Without*	*With*	*Without*
3.89	3.07	31.6	51.6	8.4	5.2

Source: Data from Leonard, R. J., & Gillis, R. (1990). Differential effects of speech prostheses in glossectomy patients (p. 705). *Journal of Prosthetic Dentistry, 64,* 701–708.

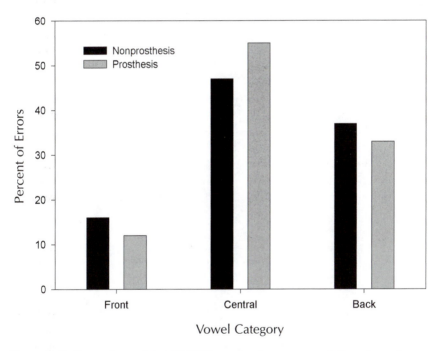

Vowel Category

Figure 7–7. Type of vowel intelligibility errors for a group of five glossectomees with and without a prosthesis. (Drawn from data presented by Leonard, R. J., & Gills, R. [1990]. Differential effects of speech protheses in glossectomy patients. *Journal of Prosthetic Dentistry, 64,* 701–708.)

CHAPTER

8

Oral Cavity Cancer Rehabilitation

I. INTRODUCTION

All previous discussions of the impact of laryngeal cancer on the individual and the family, the psychosocial needs, and the general rehabilitation considerations apply equally to the population of patients with cancers of the oral cavity. According to Myers, Barofsky, and Yates (1986):

> Centers which provide multidisciplinary patient management programs and follow adequate patient populations, thus assuring management proficiency, provide the best means of avoiding many of the pitfalls that threaten patients who are managed by a single physician and exposed sequentially to other disciplines only when problems develop. Few other cancers demonstrate the need for anticipatory treatment and rehabilitation to the magnitude required in the management of head and neck cancer. (p. 4)

Although cancers of the oral cavity constitute a small percentage of total cancers, 4% of cancers in men and 2% in women (*Oral Cancers*

Research Report, National Cancer Institute, 1988), the potential consequences of their treatment have serious implications for quality of life. The degree of disability following medical/surgical treatment will depend in large measure on the location and extent of the cancer. In a review article citing 83 references, Wells, Edwards, and Luce, (1995) stated:

A multitude of reconstructive options are possible for the patient afflicted with an intraoral malignancy. The reconstructive technique chosen depends on the stage of the disease and the extent of the soft- and hard-tissue defects after extirpation. If local tissues are not available for reconstruction, the surgeon must look to more distant sites in choosing a reconstructive procedure. Microsurgical transfer of composite tissues have allowed us a high degree of success in effecting immediate one stage closure of complex three dimensional wounds. (pg. 106)

The sequelae of this type of surgery may range from very simple to extremely complex and may include drooling, pooling of secretions, dysphagia, aspiration, changes in vocal resonance, impairment of speech production, reduction in the sense of taste, dental problems, mucosal reactions to radiation, cosmetic alterations, and psychological concerns. The optimal management of these cancers requires the highest degree of skill of the numerous health professionals who work as a coordinated team throughout the treatment process. This team should include a surgeon, medical oncologist, nurse, radiologist, speech-language pathologist, social worker, nutritionist, maxillofacial prosthodontist, and dentist. To avoid undesirable and potentially restrictive treatment outcomes and to ensure optimal long-term results, the entire team should be involved in pretreatment planning. Although the selection of treatment modality (surgery versus irradiation, radiation and chemotherapy, or other combinations) is usually dictated by the location and staging of the tumor, the choice has ramifications for resultant functional disability and for rehabilitation and its success. When surgical intervention is selected, options may exist regarding the nature and timing of surgical reconstruction and/or prosthetic replacement or augmentation. When the need for prosthetic management is anticipated, pretreatment dental assessment is essential to ensure appropriate planning for prosthesis attachment. In the majority of cases, these considerations have major ramifications for the type and severity of speech, voice, and swallowing difficulties the patient may encounter.

Appropriate pretreatment counseling of the patient requires that the kinds of treatment, their effect on functional status, and the availability and timing of rehabilitation are known by all members of the treatment team. The patient and family are then counseled in a consistent fashion.

Logemann (1994) reported the results of a prospective study of the postoperative course of 186 oral and oropharyngeal cancer patients treated surgically, many with postoperative radiotherapy. Only 50% of the patients received speech and swallowing therapy, and less than 10% received maxillofacial prosthetic intervention. At 3 months posttreatment 50% of these patients were lost to follow-up. It can be hypothesized that this particular patient sample became depressed by their functional disabilities and the lack of rehabilitation services and, in effect, gave up. This report underscores the critical need for early and active intervention of a team of specialists.

A. Incidence

According to the National Cancer Institute (*Oral Cancers Research Report*, 1988) there are an estimated 30,000 new cases of oral cancer diagnosed yearly in the United States. The U.S. Department of Health and Human Services reports that the annual age-adjusted incidence of oral cavity and pharyngeal cancers combined is 11.3 cases per 100,000. Incidence in males was almost three times that of females, and blacks had a higher rate than whites. Indeed, in black males the incidence was 24.5 per 100,000. Tongue cancer was the single largest group of oral cavity cancers accounting for almost 30% of these cases (http://www.oral-cancer.org/ profes.dir/incid.htm).

Approximately 9,000 deaths yearly are attributed to oral cancer. For combined oral cavity and pharyngeal sites, the overall mortality rate in the United States is 3.2 per 100,000. The mortality rate in males is nearly three times greater than in females, and blacks have almost twice the mortality of whites. Mortality rate for oral cavity sites alone is 1.7 deaths per 100,00. There is a higher mortality in males and in blacks (http://www.oralcancer.org). Incidence varies widely around the world.

B. Etiology

1. In the United States, the primary causes of oral cancer are tobacco use and alcohol consumption. Tobacco use of the smoked (i.e., cigarette, pipe, cigar) and smokeless varieties (i.e., chewing, dipping, sniffing) is the most common factor. Depending on the type and amount of tobacco involved, users are 4 to 15 times more likely than nonusers to develop oral cancers. Smokeless tobacco is now known to be very addictive, and in the past 20 years, its use has tripled (Spangler, 1995). Health risks clearly include oral leukoplakia and oral cancers.

2. Abuse of alcohol increases the risk of oral cancer whether or not it is associated with tobacco use. However, the effect of the combined abuse of alcohol and tobacco has a greater impact than the simple summing of their individual effects. Persons who have had one oral cancer are at increased risk for developing a new oral cancer, particularly if smoking and drinking continue to be factors.

3. Exposure to sunlight is often implicated in the etiology of lip carcinoma.

4. It is estimated that up to 60% of patients with autoimmune deficiency syndrome associated Kaposi's sarcoma (AIDS-KS) may present with the initial site of the disease in the oral cavity (Flaitz, Nicholas, & Hicks, 1995). It is also reported that most people with HIV infection will experience oral lesions at some time during the course of the disease. "Oral lesions reflect HIV status and the stage of immunosuppression, [and] are important elements in HIV staging and classification schemes" (Greenspan & Greenspan, 1996, p. 729).

5. Other factors such as dietary and metabolic deficiencies may be implicated in the etiology of oral cancers, but the evidence is not clear or definitive.

C. Diagnosis

Oral cancers may be detected visually, by palpation, or with the aid of imaging techniques (e.g., CT scan, MRI), but the diagnosis must be made by biopsy. Early detection usually results in less radical treatment procedures and, thus, more easily managed sequelae. Life expectancy is also greater following early detection and treatment.

Examination for oral cancers is often overlooked by health care providers who are too frequently remiss in detecting early oral cancers. Risk factors and signs and symptoms of early oral cancer are not generally known by the public (Horowitz, Goodman, Yellowitz, & Nourjah, 1996). Patients at high risk for oral or pharyngeal cancer, for example, smokers, heavy drinkers, and users of smokeless tobacco, should receive thorough oral examinations regularly (Mashberg & Samit, 1995).

D. Staging

All oral cancers are staged in the same manner and use the same staging system (*Oral Cancers Research Report*, 1988). Size of the tumor is indicated by the symbol T, and a numerical postscript from 1 to 4 reflects the tumor size. TX indicates a tumor that cannot be sized, TO indicates there is no evidence of a primary tumor and Tis (tumor in situ) indicates that the tumor is very small and localized to a single location. The symbol N, with a postscript of 1 to 3, is used to indicate the presence of cancer in the lymph nodes, the number involved, and the location. NX is used if the nodes cannot be assessed, and NO indicates they are free of cancer. Metastasis to distant sites is indicated by the use of MX when it cannot be determined, MO when it is absent, and M1 when it is present. Table 8–1 shows how this system is used with the four stages of cancer.

E. Treatment

1. Surgery and irradiation are the usual modalities for treatment of oral cavity cancers. Either may be used alone or in planned combination, because they have been found to complement each other. The choice of treatment modality is influenced primarily by the size and extent of the primary tumor. However, other considerations, such as morbidity, sequelae, quality of life, patient compliance, and expense must be taken into account. Chemotherapy alone or in combination with other treatments may also be used.

Table 8–1. Staging system for oral cancers.

Stage	T	N	M
I	T1 less than or equal to 2 cm	N0	M0
II	T2 2–4 cm	N0	M0
III	T3 greater than 4 cm	N0	M0
	T1, 2, or 3 of any size but not massive	N1 on same side of neck as primary	M0
IV	T4 greater than 4 cm with deep invasion	N0 or N1	M0
	Any T	N2 or N3	M0
	Any T	Any N	M1

Source: Adapted from National Cancer Institutes. (1988). *Oral Cancers Research Report* (NIH Publication Number 88-2876). Bethesda, MD: U.S. Government Printing Office.

2. Although the overall prognosis or survival of AIDS patients may not be significantly altered by treatment of oral lesions, such treatment can result in improvement in nutritional status, respiratory function, and quality of life.

F. Pretreatment Dental Assessment

This is particularly important for patients whose treatment will include radiation therapy and those for whom an intraoral prosthesis may be required.

1. Effects of radiation include a reduction in salivary flow which increases the rate of dental disease.

2. Untreated caries worsen rapidly after radiation therapy.

3. Any necessary extractions should be done prior to initiation of radiation therapy. When necessary after irradiation, extractions can put the patient at risk for serious infection, which can erode parts of the mandible.

4. Prostheses need to be anchored in order to be stable and remain in place. It is therefore important that attempts be made preoperatively to preserve critical teeth that may be needed for postoperative prosthetic stabilization. Indiscriminate extraction of essential dental units may reduce the patient's rehabilitation alternatives.

II. GLOSSECTOMY

Glossectomy refers to the surgical excision of some portion or all of the tongue. Various schemes are used to describe the extent of resection, but there is no single universally used classification system.

A. Surgical Procedures

The location, size, and extent of the tumor will dictate the amount of lingual excision that will be necessary. It must be recognized that removal of a portion of the anterior tongue is potentially much more debilitating to functions of speech and swallow than removal of an equal or greater percentage of the lateral tongue (up to 50%). An intraoral surgical approach may be feasible in cases where the lesion is very small, readily accessible, and requires minimal resection. More extensive tumors require increasingly greater resection of the tongue and adjacent structures and may necessitate splitting of the lower lip or a mandibulotomy. In the most serious cases with extensive disease, resection of the tongue, the floor of mouth, portions of the mandible, the pharynx, and the larynx may be required. Major glossectomy requires some type of surgical reconstruction.

1. Surgeons make choices about which of a variety of reconstructive techniques to use. The techniques that result in maximum mobility of the residual mass, that is, that portion of the tongue or the floor of mouth that remains following the surgery, will be the most beneficial for purposes of speech and swallowing.

2. Numerous authors have described various **reconstructive techniques** (Chowdhury, McLean, Harrop-Griffiths, & Breach, 1988; Kawashima, Harii, Ono, Ebihara, & Yoshizumi, 1989; Matloub, Larson, Kuhn, Yousif, & Sanger, 1989; Michiwaki et al., 1990; Robertson, Robinson, & Horsfall, 1987; Salibian et al., 1990; Tiwari, Greven, Karim, & Snow, 1989; Urken et al.,1991; Urken, Cheney, Sullivan, & Biller, 1995; Zieske, Johnson, Myers, Schramm, & Wagner, 1988). They include split thickness skin grafts, free radial forearm flaps, pectoralis major myocutaneous flaps, microvascular composite free flaps, free fibula grafts, and latissimus dorsi myocutaneous flaps.

B. Effects on Speech

Postoperative speech intelligibility will depend on the extent of lingual excision, the mobility of the residual tongue, the presence or absence of teeth, the type of reconstruction, as well as factors of age, hearing, general health, and motivation. The types of speech difficulties encountered can be divided into two categories: (1) articulation and (2) vocal resonance.

1. **Articulation** of speech will be affected by any impairment of lingual function. The severity of that impairment will be directly related to the site and extent of lingual resection and the degree of impedance of lingual mobility. Weakness, slowness of movement, incoordination of movement, or lack of precision of movement of the residual tongue will impede execution of the fine, precise, and rapidly coordinated sequential movements required for clear speech production. Because 17 of 25 consonants used in English rely on labiodental, linguadental, or lin-

guapalatal contact for their production, interference with this contact will have a major effect on overall clarity and intelligibility of speech. Vowel differentiations require changing the shape of the oral cavity, and the tongue plays the major role in this. Once again, inability to alter oral cavity shape adequately will further degrade the speech output.

2. **Vocal resonance** is dependent on the shape, size, and tonicity of the vocal tract. The vocal tract includes all structures above the level of the vocal folds, including the pharynx and oral cavity. Thus, alterations in vocal tract shape, size, and tonicity that occur as a result of ablative oral or oropharyngeal surgery may affect vocal resonance. The degree to which resonance is affected will depend on the extent of the surgical resection and on the nature of the reconstruction.

C. Rehabilitation of Speech

1. The speech-language pathologist should be involved in the **pretreatment planning** team meetings and should advise team members about the effects specific treatments will have on the patient's subsequent ability to communicate. Thus, when choices of type of treatment are available, consideration of their effects on communication should weigh heavily.

2. The speech-language pathologist should meet with the patient and family for a **pretreatment counseling session** to provide information about the general types of speech problems that can be anticipated. The patient should be made aware, in a broad sense, of the schedule of rehabilitation that will be followed and what professionals will be involved. It is also important that the patient and family begin to think about the role and responsibility they will have to assume in the rehabilitation process.

3. The **posttreatment counseling session** should take place when the patient no longer requires intensive care. The speech-language pathologist must be familiar with the patient's medical chart, including the operative report, to be fully aware of the extent of the surgery, the type of reconstruction, and any complications that may have been encountered. The discussion with the patient at this time will depend on the patient's overall condition and readiness, both medical and psychological, for intervention. More than a single visit may be helpful to answer the patient's and family's questions.

4. **Postoperative assessment** should take place when healing is sufficient (approximately the 7th to the 14th postoperative day or longer if complications arise) and when medical clearance has been obtained from the surgeon. The initial speech assessment should include evaluation of the oral structures, the range of motion of the tongue and jaw, oral sensation, articulation, intelligibility, and resonance.

5. **Speech treatment** should begin when it is clear that the suture lines are sufficiently healed to withstand lingual and mandibular range of motion exercises. Patients should be seen daily while they are hospitalized and weekly following discharge. The specific exercises that patients are required to do will, of course, depend on the extent of their impairment. Recalling that excision of portions of the anterior tongue are potentially more debilitating than portions of the lateral tongue, it remains that if greater than 50% of the tongue has been resected, or if there is severe limitation of movement of the residual lingual mass, range of motion exercises will be of limited value until a prosthesis has been fabricated.

   a. **Range of motion exercises** should attempt to increase vertical and anteroposterior lingual movement and lateral and horizontal movement of the mandible. The mandibular exercises are particularly important for patients who undergo irradiation following surgery. The Therabite™ Jaw Motion Rehabilitation System is a mandibular mobilization device that is engineered to encourage natural, down and back opening movements by establishing a static stretch or inducing passive motion. Mouthpiece cushions attach to the device and provide even force and firm contact with the teeth. The device, designed for single patient use, allows adjustments of the speed and range of motion by the patient within limits set by the clinician (see Appendix D for manufacturer).

   b. **Exercises to increase strength of the tongue** should focus on lateralization and elevation. Both the tip and the dorsum of the tongue should receive attention. Resistance to movement in those directions can be imposed with gradually progressive firmness using a tongue depressor as a means of increasing strength. A scale for rating lingual mobility (adapted from McConnel, Adler, & Telchgraeber, 1986) is shown in Table 8–2.

   c. Patients should be instructed in the **frequency and duration of exercise** sessions. To avoid fatigue or excessive stretching,

Table 8–2. Lingual mobility rating assessment and scale.

Tongue Position	+	–	Comments
protrude to lip			
touch upper teeth			
touch palate			
curl back			
lateralize			
right side			
left side			
depress			
front to back on palate			
Total + and – =			

Scoring: 7+ = excellent, 1 = poor

Source: Adapted from McConnel, F. M. S., Adler, R. K., & Telchgraeber, J. F. (1986). Speech and swallowing function following surgery of the oral cavity. In E. N. Myers, I. Barofsky, & J. W. Yates (Eds.), *Rehabilitation and treatment of head and neck cancer.* (NIH Publication No. 86-2762). Bethesda, MD: National Institutes of Health.

patients should be advised to practice for no longer than 2 to 3 minutes at a time approximately 5 to 10 times a day. This regimen should be continued for at least a month or more. If the patient will undergo radiation treatment following surgery, exercises should be continued through that period and for an additional 6 weeks.

d. **Attention to articulation** requires a complete analysis of sound productions. The intent should be to arrive at the most acceptable approximation of the target sound through the use of compensatory gestures rather than an attempt to recreate normal articulatory patterns. The types of compensatory gestures to be attempted must be patterned to take advantage of the patient's residual structure and the mobility of all available oral structures. Some contact between the tongue (even when reconstructed) and the palate is critical for intelligible speech. When more than 50% of the tongue has been resected, or when lingual mobility is severely reduced, attention to articulation can be delayed until the patient is fitted with an appropriate prosthetic appliance.

6. **Intraoral prosthetics** have been shown to be of value for most patients who have undergone ablative surgical procedures of the

oral cavity that resulted in a loss or immobilization of significant amounts of the tongue (Aguilar-Markulis, 1986; Leonard & Gillis, 1990; Logemann, 1989; Myer, Knudson, & Myers, 1990; Robbins, Bowman, & Jacob, 1987). Unfortunately, our understanding of the differential effects of prostheses on the speech performance of patients with different types of lingual resections is incomplete. However, in view of this inability to predict outcome, all patients deserve the opportunity to obtain improved speech through the use of an intraoral prosthesis.

7. **Fitting of intraoral prostheses.** The speech-language pathologist must work closely with the maxillofacial prosthodontist in fashioning oral prostheses. A well-fitted palate-lowering or augmentation prosthesis can make the difference between intelligible and unintelligible speech. The intent when fitting a prosthesis is to reshape the oral cavity so that the residual tongue mass may function with maximum effectiveness. Excision of portions of the tongue leaves residual spaces. The prosthesis is designed to fill those tissue defects, making contact between residual structures and the prosthesis possible at one or several points.

a. **Optimal timing** for the development of a maxillary prosthesis, whether or not the patient is to undergo a course of radiation therapy, is 4 to 6 weeks after healing is complete. This early fitting is required so that the patient does not habituate compensatory patterns that may be maladaptive. If a mandibular prosthesis is planned, its development can begin within this same time frame unless the patient will be receiving radiation therapy. In that case, it is best to postpone the development of the mandibular prosthesis until completion of irradiation.

b. **Design of the prosthesis** must be customized for the patient to fill his or her empty spaces. A number of techniques for fitting a palate augmentation prosthesis are described in the literature (Izdebski, Ross, & Roberts, 1987; Leonard & Gillis, 1990; Logemann, 1989; Myer, J.B., Jr., Knudson, R.C., & Myers, K.M., 1990). They tend to differ in small details of fitting but have much in common. The technique described here is straightforward and relies heavily on the patient's functional ability.

(1) An **acrylic base plate** is made by the prosthodontist to fit the patient's palatal contour.

(2) **Wax is added** to this base in areas where there is an absence of tissue or reduction in movement. This modeling of the base plate is done by the prosthodontist and the speech-language pathologist. The speech-language pathologist brings to this task detailed information about the patient's anatomic status, the range of movement of existing structures, and the nature of the contacts required for sound production. This information is vital in creating a model.

(3) The prosthesis is placed intraorally, and an **assessment** is made of its adequacy. The patient is asked to produce the following words and lingual movements (Logemann, 1989):

(a) tip, top, tap, two (tongue tip to alveolar ridge)

(b) chip, chop, chap, chew (tongue blade to front and midpalate)

(c) key, cap, came (midtongue to midpalate)

(d) coo, coop, cop, call (back tongue to soft palate)

(e) see, so, sue, saw (sides of tongue to lateral alveolus and narrow midline tongue groove)

(f) she, show, shoe, shop (sides of tongue to lateral alveolus and broad midline tongue groove)

(g) lingual anteroposterior sweep of the palate with the tongue as in clearing food from the palate.

(4) Based on the patient's execution of the above tasks, **wax may be added to or removed** from the base plate. If the sounds are not clear, additional wax may be required. If tongue movement is being inhibited in certain areas, removal of some wax may be necessary. This becomes a trial-and-error process, but it is not random. It is based on the patient's performance and the speech pathologist's knowledge of how sounds are produced.

(5) When an optimal level of function is achieved, the patient is instructed to **wear the prosthesis** for a week, particularly while speaking and swallowing. The wax is soft enough so that it will be molded to some extent during this process.

(6) The waxed, molded prosthesis is then **fabricated in acrylic**. The patient will continue to require speech therapy that should focus on exercises designed to habituate tongue to prosthesis placement for optimal production of speech sounds.

c. **Ratings of speech** may be made in a variety of ways. It is helpful to both the speech pathologist and the patient to chart and document performance. Ratings and assessment should be done prior to initiation of therapy, prior to introduction of a prosthesis, following the introduction of a prosthesis, during its design, and at the termination of a therapy program. Documentation of a patient's progress demonstrates progress and the outcome of speech therapy and is often required to justify continuation of funding for such therapy.

(1) A simple rating instrument is an **index of intelligibility** of speech (Allison et al., 1987) shown in Table 8–3. This index may be used by both trained and untrained listeners.

(2) **Complete phonetic analysis** of speech sound productions may provide limited information, because the nature of the compensatory sound productions may defy categorization through phonetic transcription. Therefore, a descriptive scheme that indicates the manner and place of production, a rating of the degree of accuracy, or the degree of perceptual acceptability of the affected sounds is suggested.

D. Effects on Swallow

Normal swallowing is dependent on the highly coordinated actions of the oral, pharyngeal, laryngeal, and esophageal structures.

Table 8–3. Intelligibility rating scale.

Intelligibility	Rating
No speech errors	6
Intelligible but with occasional errors	5
Intelligible but with noticeable errors	4
Intelligible with careful listening	3
Difficult to understand	2
Usually unintelligible	1

Source: Adapted from Allison et al. (1987). Adaptive mechanisms of speech and swallowing after combined jaw and tongue reconstruction in long-term survivors. *American Journal of Surgery, 154*, 419–422.

Lingual resection has a powerful effect on speech and, similarly, on deglutition. The severity of the swallowing disability is related to the extent of lingual resection, the mobility of the residual tongue, the type of reconstruction, involvement of other structures, the patient's motivation and ability to adapt, and the skill of the rehabilitation team. When more than one phase of swallowing is involved, the severity of the problem is increased. When a patient has postradiation xerostomia, specific effects on swallowing may include impaired mastication, prolonged oral phase time, and increased oral and pharyngeal residue. Complete description of the various stages of swallowing is beyond the scope of this book. The reader is referred to Logemann (1989, 1998) for further information. A complete worksheet to be used in videofluorographic swallowing evaluation is also provided by Logemann (1998).

E. Rehabilitation of Swallow

Sections C.1, C.2, and C.3 above are applicable in describing the speech-language pathologist's role in the rehabilitation team pretreatment planning and both pre- and posttreatment counseling sessions with the patient and the family by substituting the word swallow for the word speech. Therefore, they will not be repeated here. This should in no way be interpreted to imply that they are any less vital to the rehabilitation of the glossectomy patient.

1. See Section C.1, p. 196 for discussion of **pretreatment planning**.

2. See Section C.2, p. 196 for discussion of **pretreatment counseling**.

3. See Section C.3, p. 196 for discussion of **posttreatment counseling**.

4. Postoperative swallowing assessment should take place when healing is sufficient and when medical clearance has been obtained from the surgeon, about the 7th to 14th postoperative day, barring complications.

   a. The **initial assessment** may be informal and should include the following:

      (1) observation of how the patient handles his or her own secretions;

      (2) examination of the **anatomy, function, and sensory response** of the oral and pharyngeal structures;

      (3) a check for **cough, gag, and swallow reflexes**;

      (4) close observation of any **signs of aspiration**;

(5) testing the **ability to swallow** a very small amount of water and applesauce (five consecutive swallows, 5–15 ml each);

(6) assessment the patient's **readiness and motivation** for intervention;

(7) a check on the patient's **nutritional status**, which is a critical factor in decision making about the manner of feeding that should be followed.

b. The swallowing assessment should be done **prior to removal of the nasogastric feeding tube**. The tube may remain in place during the assessment.

c. When the informal testing measures, listed above, result in a clear picture that the patient is able to **swallow without aspiration and within an acceptable time frame** (10 sec or less through the oral cavity and pharynx), the nasogastric tube should be removed, and the patient should begin taking liquids and pureed foods by mouth. A skilled person (e.g., nurse, speech-language pathologist, feeding therapist) should be with the patient during the first few times when food or liquid is being taken.

d. When swallowing function appears to be disturbed, the nasogastric tube remains in place, and a complete **videofluoroscopic modified barium swallow** (with simultaneous manometry when possible) should be done and interpreted by the appropriate members of the rehabilitation team (e.g., speech-language pathologist, radiologist, nutritionist) (Logemann, 1989, 1998).

(1) The modified barium swallow will provide information about the **oral preparatory and oral swallow stages**, including the range and extent of movement of the residual tongue, how the patient is handling the preparation of the bolus, chewing, moving the bolus to the back of the mouth, clearing the oral cavity of food, and the timing of these events. In addition, it provides information on the **pharyngeal stage**, including the presence or absence of the swallowing reflex, where it is triggered, its timing, the passage of the bolus, the clearing of food from the pharynx, velopharyngeal activity, movement of the hyoid bone, and position of the larynx.

(2) **Manometry** provides information about the onset and duration of muscle relaxation, pressure changes within

the pharynx and esophagus, and their pattern during peristalsis.

e. Information derived from these studies will determine whether the patient can take **food by mouth**, what consistency the food must be, what other modes of feeding need to be used, and what type of training the patient should receive.

5. **Swallowing treatment** should begin at about the same time as speech treatment for patients who have a swallowing problem. The patient should be seen daily while in the hospital and weekly thereafter for the length of treatment required to establish swallowing with no (or minimal) aspiration at an acceptable rate of speed. The specific exercises and the nature of the compensatory movements to be taught must be determined individually and based on the type of difficulty the person is experiencing, the anatomic configuration and mobility of residual tongue, and the oral and pharyngeal sensory status. The passive, active, and resistive exercises to increase range of motion of tongue mass and jaw and to increase their strength and responsivity (see Sections 4.a, 4.b, and 4.c above) are suitable for persons who have swallowing difficulty. If these exercises are already being done for purposes of speech, additional work in those areas should not be necessary.

a. **Compensatory postures during swallowing** can be taught for a variety of reasons.
   (1) When a patient has limited antero-posterior tongue movement, **tilting the head backward** will be helpful in moving the bolus to the back of the mouth.
   (2) When the impairment is unilateral, **tilt the head to the more normal side** to take advantage of its normal function.
   (3) The **head is tilted forward** in those patients who exhibit a delayed swallow reflex to restrict the inadvertent passage of the material into the pharynx, valleculae, and airway.

b. When **less than 50% of the tongue has been excised**, and when there is some mobility remaining in the residual tongue, exercises should be devised to **encourage tongue to palate contact**.
   (1) The patient should practice **manipulating objects (food or other) in the mouth**. This involves moving the bolus in a rotary motion, positioning it between the teeth or

dental arches, and moving it from the front toward the back of the mouth. Fairly large objects, some part of which can be held by the clinician outside of the mouth, should be used first. The size of these objects can be reduced gradually.

(2) **Control of the bolus as a cohesive unit** in the mouth may also need to be practiced. Placing a small amount of paste-consistency substance on the tongue, and instruct the patient to move this around the mouth, keeping the bolus together and not allowing it to disperse in the mouth. The materials used may be expectorated without swallowing.

(3) **Food requiring chewing is introduced** in small amounts when the above activity can be done.

c. When **more than 50% of the tongue or a significant percentage of the anterior tongue has been resected, or mobility is minimal,** tongue exercises will be of little value and should be postponed until the patient is fitted with an intraoral prosthesis. However, jaw and mouth opening exercises will continue to be important, particularly for patients who undergo a course of radiation therapy.

d. If there is pharyngeal involvement that **delays triggering of the swallow reflex,** thermal stimulation of the anterior faucial pillars will be appropriate.

(1) The **technique for thermal stimulation** involves using a small size laryngeal mirror that is placed in ice water for approximately 10 sec and then gently applied to the base of the anterior faucial pillars bilaterally 5 to 10 times.

(2) This is followed by **observing and timing oral transit** time on dry swallows if the patient is restricted from taking food by mouth, or by introducing some iced water or other liquid in very small quantities at the area of the faucial arches immediately after the stimulation, if the patient can tolerate small amounts of material by mouth. The patient must be observed closely and instructed to expectorate the liquid if the swallow reflex does not operate.

(3) The **frequency and duration of thermal stimulation** depends on the patient's status. Ideally, it should be carried out numerous times during the day until the reflex triggers in under 1 sec. The reflex can be observed visu-

ally or felt by light touch of the fingers as the larynx elevates.

(4) When the swallow reflex triggers, small amounts of **liquids are introduced** in gradually increasing amounts and increasing thickness.

(5) **Severely involved patients** whose swallowing reflex fails to trigger may need extended therapy. In such cases, nonoral feeding will be required to maintain nutrition until such time as the reflex can be triggered.

e. When the **larynx is involved** either through lack of laryngeal elevation or lack of glottic closure, the patient will need to be taught the supraglottic swallow technique or the supersupraglottic swallow.

(1) In the **supraglottic swallow**, the patient is taught to hold his or her breath then swallow and release with a sharp cough immediately after the swallow. This technique is designed to close the airway before and during the swallow and then to clear residue in order to avoid any laryngeal penetration when the vocal folds open for inhalation. The extended supraglottic swallow ("dump and swallow technique") may be necessary for patients with severe reduction in tongue mobility or tongue bulk who must essentially bypass the oral transit stage of the swallow. The primary difference is that the patient must extend the neck (toss the head back) allowing gravity to drop the bolus from the mouth into the pharynx. The patient should be instructed to swallow several times while continuing to hold the breath.

(2) Some patients may benefit from exercises designed to increase glottic closure through effortful closure such as holding the breath while pressing the hands together tightly at chest height, pushing hard against a wall or down on a chair, or bearing down. This is called **the supersupraglottic swallow**. For this maneuver the patient is instructed to take a breath and hold it while bearing down, to swallow while maintaining that posture and to release with a cough. This technique attempts to tilt the arytenoids forward and produce closure of the ventricular folds as well as the true vocal folds and increase laryngeal elevation. Patients who have had a supraglottic laryngectomy or those who have had a full course of radiation therapy to the neck benefit from this technique.

f. Numerous **feeding devices** are available to assist the patient in managing feeding. These include plunger types of spoons that can be used to place the food in a particular location in the mouth, modified cups, syringes, and so forth.

g. Alternative feeding modes are required when patients are unable to manage oral feedings. These include nasogastric tube feeding, gastrostomy, orogastric tube feedings, or other long-term types of feeding tubes. Although the speech-language pathologist will have input into the need for nonoral feeding, management will be handled by nurses or caretakers, if not by the patient.

h. Intraoral prosthetics should be used for patients who have had greater than 50% of the tongue resected and/or those who have significant excision of the anterior tongue, minimal mobility of the residual lingual mass, or a reconstructed mass.

    (1) Fitting of an intraoral prosthesis is a joint activity involving the maxillofacial prosthodontist and the speech-language pathologist. The steps in fitting follow those discussed for speech purposes (see Section C.7 above). Throughout the fitting and testing stages, the patient is asked to swallow small amounts of liquid.

    (2) It is sometimes necessary to make **compromises between swallowing function and speech**. A large, bulky augmentation prosthesis may work optimally for speech, but it may impede swallow and require some reduction of its mass.

i. Surgical alternatives may be necessary in those cases in whom **intractable aspiration** persists after an appropriate trial of swallowing therapy. Total laryngectomy or an other type of surgical closure of the supraglottic respiratory tract may be necessary.

j. A **swallowing rating scale** that is fairly straightforward in determining functional status has been proposed by Sultan and Coleman (1989). This is shown in Table 8–4.

III. PALATECTOMY

Cancers of the palate may arise in the upper alveolar ridge, the hard palate, or the soft palate. The majority originate in the soft palate. The etiology of these cancers seems to be related to tobacco and alcohol use.

Table 8–4. Rating scale for swallow.

Status	Rating
No difficulty with normal diet	7
Minimal difficulty with normal diet	6
Minimal difficulty with soft diet	5
Minimal difficulty with pureed diet	4
Moderate difficulty with pureed diet	3
Severe difficulty with pureed diet	2
Inability to swallow	1

Source: Adapted from Sultan, M. R., & Coleman, J. J., III. (1989). Oncologic and functional consideration of total glossectomy. *American Journal of Surgery, 158*, 297–302.

A. Surgical Procedures

Surgical excision is usually the primary treatment of choice for cancers of the palate. Very small, localized lesions that do not invade bone may, on occasion, be treated by a course of irradiation. The location, size, and extent of the tumor will dictate the extent of surgical resection required. Of paramount importance in determining a treatment approach and prognosis is knowledge of the extent of invasion of the tumor. Staging of the tumor uses the same system described earlier.

B. Effects of Palatal Tumors on Speech and Swallow

The effect of these tumors on speech and/or swallow varies from minimal to quite severe and is highly dependent on the location of the tumor and the extent of excision.

1. Tumors of the **alveolar ridge or of the hard palate** may result in leakage of food and fluids, change in vocal resonance, distortion of some speech sounds, and difficulty chewing.

2. Tumors of the **soft palate** will affect the ability to swallow, with return of food and fluid through the nose, and will have a severe effect on vocal resonance and on the ability to produce many speech sounds. When severe, speech may be unintelligible.

C. Rehabilitation of Speech and Swallow

The speech-language pathologist plays the same role in the pretreatment planning sessions and in pre- and posttreatment counseling with the patient and family as described previously.

1. Patients with **alveolar ridge or hard palate defects** are usually fitted for an intraoral prosthesis prior to surgery, and the prosthesis is inserted at the time of surgery. This approach usually eliminates some of the effects of the surgery, allowing the patient to chew and eat without leakage and to speak with minimal alterations. Any minor speech problems remaining can usually be addressed through adaptation and habituation of compensatory behaviors.

2. Fitting of a prosthesis following excision of a **soft palate tumor** is more complex. A temporary prosthesis, without an obturating bulb extension, should be placed at the time of surgery. When healing has occurred, the prosthesis may be altered to include an obturating bulb.

3. **Videofluoroscopic examination** of the oropharynx will assist in design of the obturating bulb. The intent is to make it possible for the patient to obtain velopharyngeal closure during speech and swallow, taking full advantage of pharyngeal wall movement. This becomes more difficult if resection of the pharynx has been necessary, and the outcome for both speech and swallow may be less than optimal.

4. Some soft palate defects are being **reconstructed surgically**. Brown et al. (1997) reported that a radial forearm flap in conjunction with a superiorly based pharyngeal flap resulted in improved speech and swallow for patients requiring reconstruction of soft palate defects in which more than one quarter of the soft palate is involved.

5. **Speech assessment** should take place when sufficient healing has taken place following the surgery whether or not there has been surgical reconstruction or prosthetic management.

   a. If the **pretreatment plan did not include an intraoperative prosthesis or surgical reconstruction**, it is important to assess the patient's speech and swallow functions. Minor disturbances in these areas should receive immediate attention from the speech-language pathologist. If the problems in either area are judged to be significant and not amenable to behavioral adjustments, the speech-language pathologist must inform the rehabilitation team and make recommendations for further treatment needs.

b. If a **prosthesis was placed intraoperatively**, the speech-language pathologist should assess speech and swallowing functions several days after surgery. This assessment should determine the need for additional intervention.

c. When a **prosthesis is to be fashioned or altered postoperatively**, the speech-language pathologist should work closely with the maxillofacial prosthodontist and the radiologist to ensure that the patient's needs regarding speech and swallowing are met.

IV. MANDIBULECTOMY

A. When a tumor is located in, and restricted to, a portion of the mandible, and **excision of only a portion of the mandible** is indicated, the effects on speech and swallow are minimal. The patient often makes appropriate compensations spontaneously. Various forms of surgical reconstruction may be used as well as prosthetic devices. However, mandibular tumors that are more extensive may involve portions of the tongue and the floor of mouth (see Section II, pp. 194–207, for a discussion of glossectomy). In addition to intraoral prosthetics, discussed above, mandibular prostheses are sometimes used. These may be designed to help direct the movement of the bolus and to fill the surgically created void. They may be used singly or in conjunction with a maxillary prosthesis as long as they complement rather than interfere with each other.

B. **Mandibular reconstruction**, using a free fibula graft, can restore not only appearance, but also function. The fibula bone in the leg is cortical bone that is sufficiently long and strong enough to withstand the forces of mastication and to be a host to dental implants (Urken et al., 1995). This recent advance in surgical reconstructive technique can be extremely helpful for both speech and swallowing rehabilitation.

C. Curtis et al. (1997) reported that patients who have had **mandibular reconstruction** show better overall function and the ability to eat a more varied diet than unreconstructed patients. Improved functional ability is a major factor in quality of life issues.

V. PHARYNGECTOMY

Resection of the pharyngeal wall usually does not result in a speech problem. However, some degree of swallowing difficulty will usually result. This may be a temporary interference that will resolve as healing progresses. During this time, patients may be helped by being taught compensatory behaviors, particularly positioning to take advantage of the least impaired side. If a swallowing problem persists, it may be necessary for the patient to remain on a liquid diet and learn to handle that without aspiration.

VI. SUMMARY

"Rehabilitative surgery of the head and neck involves the most sensitive areas of the body, embracing a high aesthetic value combined with special sense organs that have many highly organized physiological functions. The combination of emotional factors and essential functional performance add a special poignancy to performing crippling surgery in this area" (Urken et al., 1995, p. xi). "The art of head and neck surgery with the diversity in reconstructive options has become a true creative endeavor" (Urken et al, 1995, p. xiii). The highest level of rehabilitation—surgical, behavioral, psychological—is the constant and ongoing focus of all those involved in the treatment of patients with head and neck cancers. New oncological methods of cancer treatment and improved surgical techniques open the way for an improved quality of life for these patients. However, they do not obviate the need for the variety of rehabilitation approaches discussed in this chapter. These approaches also undergo constant refinements and changes, and it is the responsibility of speech-language pathologists who participate in the care of head and neck cancer patients to maintain currency of knowledge and practice.

APPENDIX

A

Patient Education Materials

I. SAMPLE SCRIPT FOR PATIENT INSTRUCTION CONCERNING TEP

This is a diagram of the head and neck before the laryngectomy (see Figure 4–6). Here is the nose, the tongue, and the roof of the mouth. Here in the neck we have essentially two long tubes, or pipes. The one in the front is the trachea, or windpipe, that leads down to the lungs. The tube in the back is the esophagus that leads down to the stomach. The larynx, or voice box, sits at the top of the windpipe. The vocal folds, or vocal cords, are inside it. The larynx works as a valve, opening to let air move back and forth between the lungs and the mouth or nose as you breathe in and out. When a person speaks before laryngectomy, he or she inhales through the mouth or nose, and the larynx is open to let the air get to the lungs. Then, just as he or she is ready to speak, the vocal cords close, the air comes up from below as you start to exhale, and sets the vocal cords into vibration. The vibration becomes the sound source for speaking. As it is emitted, the articulators, the lips, tongue, teeth, and jaw, shape the sound into the various speech sounds. When you swallow, the food or liquid is in the mouth, the tongue pushes it back into the throat, and the larynx closes to keep the food and liquid out of the airway.

This is a diagram of the head and neck after the laryngectomy (see Figure 4–6). With the larynx removed, you don't have the same sound source for speaking. But also when you swallow, you don't have the larynx to protect the airway. So during the surgery, they bring the end of the windpipe out to the neck. This is the stoma that you breathe through. You can see that there's no longer a connection between the windpipe and the esophagus. So when you swallow, you don't have to worry about food "going down the wrong pipe," or "choking," because they aren't connected.

The tissue in the throat will vibrate to serve as a sound source for speaking, but you need to have air pass over it to set it into vibration. The voice restoration procedure, or tracheoesophageal puncture, creates a small tunnel through the wall that separates the windpipe from the esophagus so that air can move from the lungs into the esophagus, and start the vibration for voice. When you start to exhale, and close off the stoma, the air is directed through the tunnel or "puncture" and makes the tissue vibrate to produce a voice. Then you use your lips, tongue, teeth, and jaw to articulate the sound to make the various speech sounds. Now when you swallow, there's a problem because the food or liquid or saliva can come back through this small tunnel and fall into the lungs. That will make you cough. So you need a prosthesis to fit in the puncture to prevent this (see Figure 6–1). The prosthesis does two things. First, the prosthesis has a valve so that air can move through it to reach the esophagus and vibrate the tissue to produce voice, and the valve stays closed when you swallow so that food or liquid or saliva won't come through the puncture and down into the airway (*demonstrate the valving mechanism of the prosthesis*). The prosthesis doesn't produce the voice; it just lets air pass through it to vibrate the tissue in the throat. Second, the prosthesis keeps the tunnel or puncture open. Without something in the puncture all the way through the wall into the esophagus, either a prosthesis, a stent, or a catheter, the puncture will close back up in a matter of hours. In the meantime until it has closed, you would have problems with saliva or food or liquid leaking through the puncture into the windpipe and down to the lungs. If the puncture were to close down, you would lose your voice, because the air couldn't get through to the esophagus to vibrate the tissue. It would require another surgical procedure to recreate the puncture. So you should always have something in the puncture tract to keep it open. I'll show you how to put in a stent or catheter, so you'll always know what to do.

With the prosthesis in place, you take a breath in, close the stoma so that no air escapes through it, and then the air is directed through the prosthesis, it blows open the valve, and lets the air into the esophagus. The air makes the tissue of the throat vibrate, and this is the sound source for speaking. When you swallow, the valve stays closed, so that the food or liquid just goes past the prosthesis and down into the stomach.

II. EMERGENCY PROCEDURES

You are using an "indwelling type" prosthesis. It can only be replaced by the physician or speech pathologist.

You are using a "non-indwelling type" prosthesis. You will be instructed in how to replace this prosthesis independently.

The normal lifespan of the prosthesis will vary from a few weeks to several months depending on a variety of factors. You will know that the prosthesis needs to be replaced when:

1. it begins to leak small amounts of fluid into your stoma, causing you to cough when drinking liquids

2. voice production becomes more strained.

To check for a leak, sit in front of a mirror and shine a bright light on the prosthesis as you swallow a small amount of a colored liquid, such as coffee or grape juice. If you see drops of liquid oozing from the prosthesis, it may need replacement.

If you are using an "indwelling type" prosthesis and it begins to leak, return to your clinician for evaluation and possible replacement of the prosthesis within 24 hours or sooner. *DO NOT* attempt to replace the prosthesis yourself. If you are using a "non-indwelling type" of prosthesis and you have been instructed in how to change it you can replace it yourself.

If the voice prosthesis is accidentally dislodged from the puncture, immediately place a puncture stent (dilator) or catheter into the puncture to prevent aspiration of liquids and closure of the puncture. Keep a stent or catheter with you at all times!

In the unlikely event that prosthesis dislodgment results in aspiration (inhaling) of the voice prosthesis into the stoma, do not panic. Avoid deep inhalations, which will draw the prosthesis further into the windpipe. Bend over and attempt to cough the prosthesis out of the windpipe. If unsuccessful, seek *emergency* medical attention for removal. Most emergency room personnel are not familiar with the voice restoration technique and the prosthesis. You will need to explain to them what has happened and the necessity of keeping the dilator or catheter in the puncture. The prosthesis is radiopaque and can be seen on x-ray.

Return to your clinician if you experience any of the following:

leaking through or around the prosthesis,

difficulty achieving voice,

inflammation around the puncture site,

dislodgment of the voice prosthesis,

a prosthesis that looks too long or too short.

If you have any questions, please call your clinician at

_____ .

III. REMOVING AND REINSERTING THE VOICE PROSTHESIS

Materials: mirror   lamp   tape

               lubricating jelly   stent or catheter

               tweezers   prosthesis inserter

Preparation:

1. Wash your hands
2. Assemble supplies:

    Cut two (2) pieces of tape each 8″ long

    Cut one (1) piece of tape 1″ long
3. Sit in front of the mirror, with the light shining on your stoma. Make sure that you can see the puncture.

Procedures:

1. Using tweezers, pick off dried mucus from around the stoma and the prosthesis.
2. Put a light film of lubricating jelly on the stent/catheter.
3. Swallow—wait a few seconds.
4. Hold tab close to the prosthesis and pull it out.
5. Don't swallow.
6. Put stent/catheter in puncture and tape it securely to the neck with the two long pieces of tape.
7. Wash the prosthesis with soap and warm water, or hydrogen peroxide.
8. Check the prosthesis to make sure all residue is removed. Squeeze the prosthesis shaft to make sure that the valve is working.
9. Slide the prosthesis onto the inserter, lock the tab down.

10. Put a light film of lubricating jelly on the prosthesis.

11. Swallow—wait a few seconds.

12. Remove the stent/catheter; don't swallow.

13. Line the prosthesis up with the puncture.

14. Insert the prosthesis, feel it pop into place.

15. While still attached to the inserter, gently rotate the prosthesis 360°. It should turn freely if it is fully inserted. If it is not properly inserted, repeat steps 4–15.

16. Lift the tab off the inserter, slide inserter out of the prosthesis while holding on to the tab.

17. Use the small piece of tape to secure the tab to the skin.

Note: If you have trouble inserting the prosthesis, replace the stent/catheter, wait several minutes, and try again.

Always keep a stent/catheter in the puncture when the prosthesis is not in place. Otherwise, saliva and food will leak into your windpipe and the puncture will close.

IV. TRACHEOSTOMA ("HANDS-FREE") VALVE

Valve Attachment

1. Make sure the prosthesis is properly inserted and the voice is adequate.

2. Clean the skin area surrounding the stoma with soap and water. Let dry.

3. Sit in front of a well-lighted mirror.

4. Hold the housing up to the stoma to visualize the area that will be covered.

   a. If the area is irregular, flatten it out using your hands or extend the neck.

   b. Cut the tab of the prosthesis to meet the outer edge of the housing on a standard prosthesis (Indwelling prostheses usually already have the tab removed). For a standard prosthesis, DO NOT CUT BEYOND THE HOLE ON THE TAB; this is needed for locking the insertion tool onto the prosthesis.

5. Apply a skin barrier (e.g., Shield Skin™ or Skin Prep™). Avoid dripping into the stoma.

6. A thin film of glue will be placed around the stoma corresponding to the size of the housing. (*Note:* Glue will not come out of clothing!) Remove the brush and scrape its entire length along the inside of the bottle to remove any excess. Dip only the brush portion into the glue. Begin applying to the skin. Pay extra attention to suture lines and skin folds to make sure that they are adequately covered. Be certain to not allow any glue to get into the stoma!

7. Place a small amount of glue on both sides of the prosthesis tab (non-indwelling prosthesis).

8. Let the glue dry for 4 minutes (use a stopwatch).

9. While the glue is drying, prepare the housing. Take a clear tape disc and peel off the backing on one side. Avoid finger or surface contact with the adhesive tape discs and foam discs to prevent loss of adherence. The easiest way to hold it is to place your index finger inside the opening and your thumb on the outside edge.

10. Place the housing back (flat) side up on a firm surface. Shape it convexly, so that the sides are pointed downward.

11. (Optional tape disc placement) Remove the paper backing from one side of the tape disc. Line up the opening of the tape disc with the housing, exposed adhesive side down. Using your fingers, start with the center, and press the tape disc onto the housing. As you work toward the edges, shape the housing concavely, so that the sides are pointed up. Smooth out the air bubbles as much as possible. Remove the second backing from the tape disc. Place the housing on the firm surface, convexly, with the adhesive side up.

12. Remove the paper backing from one side of the foam disc. Line up the opening of the foam disc with the housing, exposed adhesive side down. Using your fingers, start with the center, and press the foam disc onto the housing. As you work toward the edges, shape the housing concavely, so that the sides are pointed up. Smooth out the air bubbles as much as possible. Remove the second backing from the foam disc.

13. Using the wooden end of a cotton-tipped applicator, press the prosthesis tab against the skin. Place housing up to the designated area around the stoma. Flatten neck out before placing.

14. Press the housing to the neck, beginning with "problem areas" such as suture lines or skin folds. Groove and bend the housing to get a good seal. Work all areas from inner area toward the edges.

Adjustable Valve Placement

1. Turn the valve handle to set the correct opening as described below.

2. Place one hand on the housing to help hold it in place against the neck. To insert the valve into the housing, hold the valve by the edge (not the bar), and line up the valve with the bottom of the housing opening. Use the valve to stretch the opening downward and roll it in toward the top.

3. Begin voice production. To get the valve to close, it will take a rapid blast of air. After the valve closes, you can let up on the pressure until you find the minimum amount of effort needed to keep the valve closed. Adjust the setting of the valve as necessary. It should be open enough that breathing is easy, but not so much that it requires extreme effort to get it to snap shut for voice production.

4. Take a short walk and re-set the valve as needed.

5. If the silicone flapper blows out, push it back in. It must be curled around the hook to work properly.

6. To remove the valve, place a finger on the housing to keep it in place. Use the other hand to grasp the edge (not the handle) of the valve and pull it open like a door from right to left.

7. Remove the valve, leave the housing in place if you sense a cough starting. Wipe inside the housing and around the stoma thoroughly. Secretions will break the adhesive seal prematurely. If secretions are excessive, consider a heat and moisture exchange (filter) system.

8. During increased physical activity, you may want to open the valve slightly more to allow for a deeper inhalation.

9. Do not sleep with the valve in. Do not leave the housing attached for longer periods than recommended by the manufacturer as the skin may become irritated.

10. After removing the housing, clean the skin with warm water and soap. Do not rub as it may cause irritation. If the glue is

difficult to remove, consider using some of the adhesive remover pads (e.g., Remove™) available from the prosthesis supply companies. Be careful not to allow these products to drip into your stoma.

11. If you are using a reusable housing which is not self-adherent: To remove the adhesive backing from the housing, begin at one edge and roll the backing loose with your thumb. The use of the clear tape discs helps in the removal. Wash the housing with warm water and soap. (Do not use rubbing alcohol as it will stiffen the housing.) Allow it to dry thoroughly before attempting to attach new adhesives.

It takes practice and patience to be successful with the hands-free valve. The use of minimum respiratory effort is critical to reducing the "back pressure" that contributes to premature loss of a seal. With repeated applications, the likely location of adhesive seal breaks will be obvious. Pay particular attention to these areas when applying the adhesive prior to attachment.

V. CARE OF THE LARYNGECTOMIZED PATIENT IN THE HOSPITAL

1. This patient is a neck breather and is not able to produce normal voice.

2. The patient may have learned a different way to talk. Find out about it.

   a. The patient may use an electronic speech aid or may have a prosthesis in place to assist in producing speech.

   b. Another possibility is that the patient has learned esophageal speech for which no devices are necessary.

3. If the patient is very ill these forms of speech may be too difficult to use. A communication board of some type might be useful.

4. Due to anatomic changes, the patient cannot blow his or her nose.

5. When the patient coughs, mucus may be blown out of the stoma. Stoma coverings can be very useful and need to be kept moist.

6. It is helpful to keep the humidity in the room up to 50%.

7. Oxygen requires the use of a nebulizer and a special tracheostomy collar. Drain the nebulizer hose frequently by disconnecting it from the tracheostoma collar first. Do not lift the hose or allow the condensation to pour into the stoma.

8. Frequent position changes and extra humidification are helpful in avoiding pneumonia and other respiratory complications.

9. Use a warm, moist cloth to wipe the stoma area once or twice a day to avoid crusting or to remove dried secretions.

10. In the event of irritation of the skin surrounding the stoma, always use a water-based ointment or lotion. Avoid the use of petroleum-based products which can be inhaled and cause pneumonia.

11. Shaving and hair care should be done only when the stoma cover is in place.

12. A special laryngectomy shower collar should be used when showering. If not available, a face cloth should be held lightly over the stoma.

13. Respond quickly to the call light—the patient cannot shout.

14. Learn the special CPR techniques of mouth/mask to stoma breathing. Patients using the internal prosthesis for speech (tracheoesophageal puncture—TEP) must have both mouth and nose totally sealed during CPR.

15. If the patient uses a prosthesis (TEP), find out about its care.

    a. Indwelling prostheses may be left in place, but the others need to be removed, cleaned, and re-inserted.

    b. It is important that the puncture site not be left unfilled for more than a few minutes by either a prosthesis or a catheter.

16. Do not shout, use baby talk, or exaggerated speech when talking to a laryngectomee. They can hear and understand but have difficulty speaking.

APPENDIX

B

Problem Solving for TEP

FLEXIBLE VIDEOENDOSCOPIC VERIFICATION OF THE VOICE PROSTHESIS

1. The clinician should have received requisite training specifically in the method of flexible endoscopy.

2. A topical anesthetic can be administered by qualified medical professionals, as necessary, to reduce patient discomfort. Ideally, topical anesthesia should be limited to viscous lidocaine to ease the passage of the flexible endoscope through the nasal passages, as excessive oropharyngeal secretions associated with the use of anesthetic sprays will reduce visualization of structures.

3. Using a constant light source, the scope is advanced through the nasal passage and into the pharynx.

4. If copious pooled secretions are present, the patient should drink a small amount of warm water to clear the pharyngoesophagus for visualization.

5. At this point, the patient is asked to dry swallow slowly as the examiner gently advances the scope into the esophagus. In some laryngectomees, an "esophageal bar" may be visible which divides the pharyngoesophagus in the AP dimension. Care should be taken to enter the esophagus posteriorly to the bar, as anteriorly the pharynx will terminate in a blind pocket. Esophageal perforation may result from advancement of the scope into this diverticulum.

6. The scope is advanced inferiorly to a level that is just below the puncture site in the esophagus. Orientation as to the vertical level of the scope is facilitated by observing the location of the light on the exterior of the patient's neck.

7. The patient is asked to occlude the stoma and produce a soft prolonged /a/. As the patient phonates, the examiner should slowly retract the scope until it is at a level slightly above the prosthesis. Several attempts may be necessary to position the scope properly for adequate visualization, requiring advancement of the scope to a level below the prosthesis and retraction with prolonged phonation.

8. If the prosthesis cannot be visualized during phonatory tasks, the above procedure should be repeated while the patient attempts a "slow" dry swallow manuever.

9. When properly placed, the esophageal retention collar of the prosthesis should be fully open into the lumen of the esophagus (see Figure 6–4). If the prosthesis is not fully inserted into the esophagus, only a shadow of the prosthesis or a bulging of the mucosa may be visible (see Figure 6–4).

10. Following visualization, the endoscope is gently withdrawn.

PROBLEM-SOLVING GUIDE

Problem	Possible Cause	Solution
Difficulty inserting prosthesis	⇨ Puncture closing	⇨ Dilate with stent or catheter
	⇨ Low pressure prosthesis	⇨ Use duckbill or gel cap
	⇨ Angled puncture	⇨ Use catheter to check angle, direct inferiorly; Re-puncture
	⇨ Puncture difficult to visualize	⇨ Pull up skin to visualize; Recline patient
	⇨ Resistance	⇨ Dilation; Use lubricant
Painful insertion	⇨ Prosthesis not fully inserted	⇨ Remove, dilate and re-insert
	⇨ TE tract stenosis	⇨ Dilate and re-insert
	⇨ GE reflux	⇨ Anti-reflux protocol
	⇨ Granulation tissue, irritation	⇨ Dilate 1–2 sizes larger than prosthesis, then insert; Cauterize
Microstoma	⇨ Stenosis	⇨ Fenestrated laryngectomy tube; Surgical revision
Macrostoma	⇨ Natural tracheal size; Tracheomalac	⇨ Surgical revison
Immediate post-fitting aphonia; effortful phonation	⇨ "Overfitting" prosthesis (too long)	⇨ Remove prosthesis and resize
	⇨ Valved tip is closed	⇨ Flush in situ with pipette; Remove prosthesis, inspect, squeeze end
	⇨ Forceful stoma occlusion	⇨ Lighten finger contact with downward pressure

(continued)

Problem	Possible Cause	Solution
Immediate post-fitting aphonia; effortful phonation (*continued*)	⇨ Post/radiation edema (primary puncture and early secondary punctures)	⇨ Replace catheter, allow edema to subside (up to 4 weeks), refit
	⇨ Pharyngeal constrictor hypertonicity/spasm	⇨ Assess voicing "open tract"; Transtracheal insufflation via 18-Fr catheter; Pharyngeal plexus nerve block; Insufflate under fluoroscopy; If confirmed, consider myotomy or Botox™ injection
	⇨ Excessive resistance	⇨ Change to low pressure or 20-Fr. prosthesis
	⇨ Gel cap has not dissolved	⇨ Drink water, wait 4 minutes
Delayed post-fitting aphonia	⇨ Valve tip is closed	⇨ Flush in situ with pipette; Remove prosthesis, inspect, squeeze end
	⇨ Puncture tract closure due to "underfitting"	⇨ Dilate, resize, insert longer prosthesis; Repuncture
	⇨ Prosthesis not fully inserted	⇨ Dilate and re-insert; Confirm with endoscopy or radiographic study
	⇨ False tract creation associated with re-insertion of prosthesis	⇨ Replace catheter and re-insert; Confirm with endoscopy or radiographic study
Leakage through prosthesis	⇨ Valve deterioration	⇨ Replace prosthesis
	⇨ Candida deposits	⇨ Disinfect prosthesis with hydrogen peroxide; Nystatin suspension
	⇨ Duckbill tip against posterior pharyngeal wall	⇨ Resize; Replace with correct size; Replace with low pressure prosthesis
		⇨ Repeated dry swallows; flush in situ
	⇨ Valve is stuck in the open position due to food or saliva	⇨ Use wooden tip of cotton applicator to gently release the valve

	⇧ Valve is stuck in the open position immediately post-insertion	⇧ Dilate for longer period of time before prosthesis insertion
	⇧ Post-insertion kinking of prosthesis causing valve to stay in the open position	
	⇧ Resistance of flap valve too low	⇧ Place duckbill or high resistance prosthesis
Leakage around prosthesis	⇧ Overfitting; prosthesis pistons in tract	⇧ Resize; Replace with correct size prosthesis; Consider retention collar for in-between sizes
	⇧ Tract dilation in irradiated tissue	⇧ Place smaller catheters (10–12 Fr.); Place prosthesis of soft silicone; Use larger retention collar; Flap reconstruction
	⇧ Tract dilation due to plaque deposits	⇧ Replace prosthesis more frequently
	⇧ Superior migration of tract resulting in vertical positioning of prosthesis	⇧ Replace catheter and direct inferiorly; Allow tract to close and re-puncture
	⇧ Insufficient party wall thickness	⇧ Reconstruct with muscle flap
Dislodgment of prosthesis	⇧ Prosthesis not fully inserted	⇧ Resize and re-insert; Retrain or consider extended wear prosthesis
	⇧ Poor condition of tissue causing tract dilation	⇧ See under "Leakage around prosthesis"; Muscle flap
	⇧ Forceful cough	⇧ Consider extended wear prosthesis
Granulation Tissue	⇧ Irritation associated with presence of foreign body	⇧ Surgical removal of tissue; Cauterization
	⇧ Inflammation from infrequent removal of prosthesis	⇧ Retrain; Regularly rotate prosthesis in tract

(continued)

231

Problem	Possible Cause	Solution
Frequent belching; gastric air	⇨ Pharyngoesophageal stricture	⇨ Mechanical dilation; Surgical revision
	⇨ Pharyngeal constrictor hypertonicity/spasm	⇨ Myotomy or chemical denervation
	⇨ Prosthesis opening due to pressure changes	⇨ Change to duckbill or high resistance prosthesis
	⇨ Hypotonic PE segment	⇨ Pressure band to the PE segment
	⇨ GI dysfunction	⇨ Refer to GI
Inability to digitally occlude stoma	⇨ Irregular stoma configuration	⇨ Custom adaptive devices; Fit with tracheostoma valve; Surgical revision
	⇨ Upper extremity dysfunction	⇨ Adaptive devices; Fit with tracheostoma valve
Poor quality speech	⇨ Prosthesis not fully inserted	⇨ Remove, resize and place correct prosthesis
	⇨ Loose segment, esp. with pharyngeoesophageal reconstructions	⇨ Digital pressure; Pressure band; Manual occlusion instead of tracheostoma valve
	⇨ Tight segment, poor elasticity of segment	⇨ Reduce effort; Change to low pressure or 20 Fr. prosthesis; Moisture
	⇨ Poor vibratory activity	⇨ Change to low resistance or 20 Fr. prosthesis; Alter tone focus; Retrain stoma occlusion
	⇨ Air leakage around stoma	⇨ Retrain stoma occlusion; Adaptive devices; tracheostoma valve
	⇨ Short phrases	⇨ Reduce effort; Change to 20 Fr or low resistance prosthesis; retrain respiratory effort
	⇨ Strained high pitch	⇨ Alter tone focus to lower in throat
	⇨ Excessively low pitch	⇨ Alter tone focus higher in throat

Insufficient duration of tracheostoma valve seal

⇧ Excessive "back pressure"

⇧ Assess with pressure meter during speech; Change to 20-Fr or low resistance prosthesis; Reduce loudness/effort; Consider change to Barton-Mayo button

⇧ Inadequate cleansing of skin prior to application

⇧ Remove old adhesive completely with Remove™; Use SkinPrep™ or alcohol to prepare area

⇧ Failure to allow adhesive to set

⇧ Wait four minutes for adhesive to dry before applying housing; Use self-adhering housings

⇧ Careless application of tape and foam discs to housing

⇧ Retrain application procedures to remove air bubbles; Use self-adhering housings

⇧ Irregular peristomal area configuration

⇧ Retrain application method with extra care to irregular area; Use larger self-adhering housings; Pull up and smooth skin before application; Attempt use of skin barrier products to form more regular area; Custom housing for tracheostoma valve; Consider change to Barton-Mayo button

⇧ Break in seal due to secretions

⇧ Remove valve prior to cough, wipe secretions carefully from inside surface of housing chimney; Consider heat-moisture exchange system (e.g., Humidifilter™); prescription medications (Ponaris™)

233

APPENDIX

C

Support and Referral Organizations

This listing is very basic and does not include local groups. The speech-language pathologist should become aware of all groups within his or her geographic area that provide services to the laryngectomized population.

The International Association of Laryngectomees (IAL)
7440 N. Shadeland Avenue, Suite 100
Indianapolis, IN 46250

The International Association of Laryngectomees (ILP) is the overall, umbrella group and has member groups in many communities. The IAL can inform the speech-language pathologist about affiliated groups within any given geographic area. The IAL publishes a newsletter three times yearly that is available to all laryngectomized individuals, as well as to speech-language pathologists. The IAL sponsors an annual Voice Institute and an Annual Meeting which provide an opportunity for laryngectomees, their families, and speech-language pathologists to come together for learning and recreation. The IAL prints a directory of certified alaryngeal speech instructors.

The American Cancer Society
1599 Clifton Road, NE
Atlanta, GA 30329

There are state divisions of the American Cancer Society as well as regional offices. They can usually be found in the local telephone directory. The American Cancer Society, in addition to providing information kits, can be a valuable resource for locating local support groups and making films and various publications available. In some localities, they may loan pieces of equipment and offer various other types of support to persons with cancer.

The American Speech-Language-Hearing Association
10801 Rockville Pike
Rockville, MD 20852

The American Speech-Language-Hearing Association (ASHA) can provide speech-language pathologists with guidance and direction about professional practices. Guidelines and Position Papers are useful in delineating the Scope of Practice of the speech-language pathologist with laryngectomized and head and neck cancer populations (see *Guidelines for Evaluation and Treatment for Tracheoesophageal Fistulization/ Puncture*. ASHA, 1992), as well as indicating the skills necessary to be proficient in providing the services. ASHA can direct patients to sources of available services within their geographic area.

APPENDIX

D

Suppliers and Manufacturers

PNEUMATIC AND ELECTRONIC SPEECH AIDS, AMPLIFIERS, BATTERIES, AND ACCESSORIES

Artificial Speech Aids: Westridge Acres, 3001-8 12th Street, Harlan, IA 51537
Phone and fax: (712) 755-2389
Tokyo Artificial Larynx (Pneumatic) and accessories

A.S Telecom, Inc: 9915 Saint Vital St., Montreal, Quebec, H1H 4S5 Canada
Phone: (514) 326-5423; Fax: (514) 326-6576
Romet, Cooper-Rand, Denrick, Nu-Vois, Vocaltech, batteries, accessories, repairs

Audiphone Company of South Texas:
711 Navarro, Ste 204, San Antonio, TX 78205
Phone: (210) 223-2033; Toll-Free (800) 683-3277
Servox and accessories

Band K Prescription Shop: 601 East Iron, Salina, KS 67401
Phone: (913) 827-4455; Toll-Free (800) 432-0224
Servox, batteries, accessories

Tom Beneventine: 58 Woodstock Dr., Wayne, NJ 07407
Phone: (201) 694-8417
Servox, batteries, accessories

Bruce Medical Supply:
411 Waverly Oaks Rd., P.O Box 9166, Waltham, MA 02254
Phone: (617) 894-6262; Toll-Free: (800) 225-8446; Fax: (617) 894-9519
Servox, Bruce Electrolarynx, Batteries

California Speech and Hearing Instruments:
1930 Wilshire Blvd. #810, Los Angeles, CA 90057
Phone: (213) 483-4481; Fax: (213) 483-0527
Cooper-Rand, Neovox, Servox, Macrovox, Romet, Nu-Vois, batteries,
amplifiers, repairs

Care Medical Supply: 2 Harvey St., Rome, GA 30161
Phone: (706) 232-2001; Toll-Free: (800) 273-1763
Servox Inton, batteries, amplifiers, accessories

Communicative Medical, Inc: P.O. Box 8241, Spokane, WA 99203-0241
Phone: (509) 838-1060; Toll-Free: (800) 944-6801
Servox, Nu-Vois,Trutone, Solatone, Toneaire (pneumatic), Romet, chargers,
batteries, intraoral adapters, amplifiers, repairs, reconditioned artificial larynges,
and more

Freeman's Hearing Aid Center:
2230 E. Pikes Peak Ave., Colorado Springs, CO 80909
Phone: (719) 632-2376
Servox and accessories

Jessie Hart: 1750 Avenue East, Grand Prairie, TX 75051
Phone: (214) 264-3129
Servox, Romet, SPKR, NuVois, batteries and accessories

Griffin Laboratories: 27636 Ynez Rd., Temecula, CA 92591
Phone: (909) 698-5451; Fax: (909) 698-3040
TruTone

Health Concepts, Inc: 279-B Great Valley Parkway, Malvern, PA 19355
Phone: (215) 889-7363: Toll-Free: (800) 721-4848
UltraVoice

InHealth Technologies: 1110 Mark Ave., Carpinteria, CA 93013-2918
Phone: (805) 684-9337; Toll-Free: (800) 477-5969; Fax: (805) 684-8594
Servox, batteries

International Medical Resources Industries (IMRI):
P.O. Box 120, Brookfield, CT 06804-0120
Phone: (203) 775-6366; Fax: (202) 775-0522
Batteries, Servox, Romet

Jack Kemp Enterprises: 44547 Woodrow Way, Hemet, CA 92544
Phone: (909) 927-7534; Toll-Free: (800) 735-2922; Fax: (909) 927-5871
TruTone

Kenneth W. Jansen: 9407 Catalina Drive, Brandenton, FL 34210
Phone: (813) 792-4251
Romet and Servox

Lakewood Hearing and Speech Center:
3110 S. Wadsworth, Ste 107, Lakewood, CO 80227
Phone: (303) 988-7299
Servox and accessories

Lauder Enterprises: 11115 Whisper Hollow, San Antonio, TX 78230-3609
Phone: (210) 492-1984; Toll-Free: (800) 388-8642; Fax: (210) 492-0864
Servox, Nu-Vois, Denrick, Romet, PO Vox, Trutone, batteries, chargers,
amplifiers, repairs, and more.

Luminaud, Inc: 8688 Tyler Blvd, Mentor, OH 44060
Phone: (440) 255-9082; Fax: (440) 255-2250
Nu-Vois, Denrick 2, Cooper-Rand, Tru-Tone, SolaTone, amplifiers,
publications, accessories

Memacon: P.O. Box 56, 6880 AB Velp, The Netherlands
Phone: (0) 85-618708
DSP 8 Pneumatic artificial larynx

Park Surgical Company: 5001 New Utrecth Ave, Brooklyn, NY 11219
Phone: (718) 436-9200; Toll-Free: (800) 633-7878
Bruce Electronic Artificial Larynx, amplifiers

Professional Hearing & Speech Aids: 30 Salem Market Pl., Salem, CT 06103
Phone: (203) 525-2131 or (203) 859-2807; Fax: (203) 859-3102
Servox, Romet, Cooper-Rand, Nu-Vois, and amplifiers

Romet, Inc: 929 SW Higgins Avenue, Missoula, MT 59803
Phone: (406) 251-5568; Fax: (406) 251-5570
Romet Electrolarynx and oral adapters

Dean Rosecrans: P.O. Box 310, Nampa, ID 83653-0310
Phone: (208) 467-4790; Toll-Free: (800) 522-4425;
Toll-Free: (800)237-3699 (Canada/Mexico)
SPKR, Varta Battery

Siemens Hearing Instruments, Inc:
16 East Piper Ln., Ste 128, Prospect Heights, IL 60070
Toll-Free: (800) 333-9083; Fax: (708) 808-1299
Servox, batteries, and accessories

Slobodian Enterprises: 345 Milpond Dr., San Jose, CA 95126
Phone: (408) 297-3469
Romet, Servox, Nu-Vois, SPKR, batteries

Synergistic Batteries, Inc: 3760 Lower Roswell Rd., Marietta, GA 30068
Phone: (404) 973-2220; Toll-Free: (800) 634-600
Servox and Romet Batteries

UltraVoice: 19 E. Central Ave, Paoli, PA 19301
Toll-Free: (800) 721-4848
UltraVoice Intra-Oral Speech Aid

Uni Mfg Co.: P.O. Box 607, Ontario, OR 97914
Phone: (503) 889-6567; Toll-Free: (800) GET-SPKR
SPKR

Unipower: 1216 W. 96th St, Minneapolis, MN 55431
Phone: (612) 884-2933; Toll-Free: (800) 542-6998; Fax: (612) 884-1726
Servox, batteries

VOICE PROSTHESES, HEAT/MOISTURE EXCHANGERS, SUPPLIES AND THERAPY AIDS

Atos Medical AB: PO Box 183, S-242 22 Horby, Sweden
Phone: (46) 415-17600
Provox Voice Restoration System, Provox Stomafilter

Bio Med Prosthetics: R.R. 1 Box 740, Brooks, ME 04921
Phone: (207) 722-3462; Toll-Free: (800) 824-2492; Fax: (207) 722-3320
Special prosthetics for cosmetic and speech problems

Bivona, Inc: 5700 West 23 Ave, Gary, IN 46406
Phone: (219) 989-9150; Toll-Free: (800) 348-6064; Fax: (219) 844-9031
Bivona Colorado Voice Restoration System, Bivona Duckbill Prosthesis,
Bivona Ultra-low Resistance Voice Prosthesis, Optivox, Tracheostoma Vents,
Tracheostoma Valves and Kits, Provox Voice Restoration System, Provox
Stomafilter, Stom-vent/Stom-vent 2, accessories

Bruce Medical Supply:
411 Waverly Oaks Rd., P.O Box 9166, Waltham, MA 02254
Phone: (617) 894-6262; Toll-Free: (800) 225-8446; Fax: (617) 894-9519
Double-sided adhesive foam disks for Bivona and Blom-Singer tracheostoma
valves

E. Benson Hood Laboratories, Inc:
5757 Washington St., Pembroke, MA 02359
Phone: (617) 826-7573; Toll-Free: (800) 942-5227; Fax: (617) 826-3899
Panje Voice Prosthesis, tracheostoma valves

InHealth Technologies: 1110 Mark Ave., Carpinteria, CA 93013-2918
Phone: (805) 684-9337; Toll-Free: (800) 477-5969; Fax: (805) 684-8594
Blom-Singer Duckbill and Low Pressure Voice Prosthesis, Indwelling
Prostheses, Blom-Singer Tracheostoma Valves, Blom-Singer Laryngectomy
Tubes, Blom-Singer HumidiFilter, Accessories and supplies

THERAPY AIDS

The Therabite Corporation:
4661 West Chester Pike, Newtown Square, PA 19073-2227
Phone: (610) 356-9500 ; Toll-Free: (800) 322-2650

AMPLIFIER SUPPLIERS

California Speech and Hearing Instruments:
1930 Wilshire Blvd. #810, Los Angeles, CA 90057
Phone: (213) 483-4481: Fax: (213) 483-0527
Macrovox, Voicette

Communicative Medical, Inc: P.O. Box 8241, Spokane, WA 99203-0241
Phone: (509) 838-1060; Toll-Free: (800) 944-6801
Piper-1 Personal Amplifier and adapter

Lauder Enterprises: 11115 Whisper Hollow, San Antonio, TX 78230-3609
Phone: (210) 492-1984; Toll-Free: (800) 388-8642; Fax: (210) 492-0864
Flex Mike and Mini Vox amplifiers

Luminaud, Inc.: 8688 Tyler Blvd, Mentor, OH 44060
Phone: (440) 255-9082; Fax: (440) 255-2250
Rand Voice Amplifier (pocket size), Voicette Amplifier, Mini Vox Amplifier,
and Texas Instrument Vocaid

Park Surgical Company: 5001 New Utrecth Ave, Brooklyn, NY 11219
Phone: (718) 436-9200; Toll-Free: (800) 633-7878
Speech amplifier with headset, Speech amplifier with throat microphone,
Extension Speaker, Pausaid, and Loudness Indicator

Professional Hearing & Speech Aids: 30 Salem Market Pl., Salem, CT 06103
Phone: (203) 525-2131 or (203) 859-2807; Fax: (203) 859-3102
Flex Mike Amplifier, Rand amplifier, Vocaid, Voicette Amplifier, Speechmaker
Amplifier

Stanton Magnetics, Inc: 101 Sunnyside Blvd, Plainview, NY 11803
Phone: (516) 349- 0235; Toll-Free: (800) 526-3684; Fax: (516) 349-0230
ADDvox-Bone conduction amplifier/speaker system with head band or neck
band microphone and accessories. ADDvox Bullhorn bone conduction speech
projection system with head band or neck band microphones and accessories.

APPENDIX

E

Contents of a Laryngectomee Kit

There is no single standard laryngectomee kit. The contents vary by state and by locality. Because kits are usually provided by the American Cancer Society, their contents may be dependent on the presence of an active rehabilitation and service committee with members who are up-to-date in their knowledge of the needs of the laryngectomized individual. We urge speech-language pathologists (SLPs) to become involved with their local Cancer Society and offer assistance in reviewing the currency of laryngectomee kit contents.

The following is a listing of some things we have found to be helpful and which could form the core of a laryngectomee kit.:

   1. Bright orange EMERGENCY ID cards to be carried by the patient and to affix to the car windshield.

   2. *First Aid for Laryngectomees* and its Supplement. This is a publication of the American Cancer Society.

3. A recent copy of the *IAL* (International Association of Laryngectomees) News.

4. Pamphlets on Home Care Information on Tracheostomy Tube Care and Suctioning the Tracheostomy produced by the Roswell Park Memorial Institute.

5. Single sheets of information as follows:

   a. Methods of Speech Following Laryngectomy provides short descriptions of all available methods.

   b. Hints for Families and Friends

   c. Hints for Hygiene and Grooming

   d. Instructions for making crocheted stoma covers

6. A brochure about MedicAlert.

7. A listing of local sources of help which can be completed by the speech-language pathologist or the patient.

8. A copy of *Self-Help for the Laryngectomee*, by Edmund Lauder, edited by James Lauder.

A P P E N D I X

F

LARYNGECTOMEE CASE HISTORY
AND ASSESSMENT FORM

Syracuse Voice Center
SUNY Health Science Center, Syracuse NY

Name: _____ DOB:_____

Evaluation Date: _____

Address: _____

Phone: (   ) _____ Referred by:_____

MEDICAL HISTORY:

Primary site of tumor: _____ ICD9: _____ Surgery date: _____

Staging: T: _____ N: _____ M: _____ Surgeon:_____

Prelaryngectomy Rx: ☐ none ☐ radiation ☐ chemotx ☐ prior surgery (specify

procedure and date)_____

Extent of surgery: ☐ partial laryngectomy ☐ total laryngectomy ☐ myotomy

☐ pharyngectomy ☐ esophagectomy ☐ partial anterior glossectomy

☐ partial lateral glossectomy ☐ <50% ☐ >50%

☐ neck dissection: ☐ unilateral ☐ bilateral ☐ standard ☐ modified

Closure/reconstruction: ☐ primary ☐ free flap ☐ jejunal ☐ gastric pullup

☐ other (describe)_____

Complications: (describe)_____

TEP: ☐ primary ☐ secondary (date: _____)

Post op Radiotx: #treatments_____ #Rads_____ Date completed:_____

General Health: (other conditions, other surgeries):_____

_____

Medications:_____

SOCIAL/OCCUPATIONAL HISTORY:

Occupation:_____

Do you plan to return to work? ☐ same job ☐ different job ☐ no

With whom do you live? _____

Family/friends adjustment?_____

CURRENT STATUS:

Hearing: ☐ unaided ☐ aided ☐ untested: self-appraisal: ☐ ok ☐ problem

Vision: ☐ glasses ☐ no glasses; self-appraisal: ☐ ok w/glasses ☐ problem

Dental: ☐ edentulous ☐ full dentures ☐ other (describe)_____

Swallowing:(describe any

difficulties)_____

Chewing:_____Taste:_____ Smell:_____

Tongue: range of motion:_____

Reconstruction or prosthesis:_____

Cognitive status:_____ Emotional status:_____

Prior voice/speech rehab: (describe)_____

Primary communication: ☐ writing ☐ artificial larynx (type): _____

☐ TEP ☐ esophageal ☐ other _____

Secondary communication: ☐ writing ☐ artificial larynx (type)_____

☐ TEP ☐ esophageal ☐ other _____

For TE prosthesis users only: style & size of prosthesis:_____

date fitted:_____ **date placed:**_____ **Tracheostoma valve** ___**yes**___**no**

PROGNOSIS FOR ACQUISITION OF:

Electronic/mechanical speech:_____

Esophageal speech:_____

Tracheoesophageal speech:_____

Independent prosthesis management skills:_____

RECOMMENDATIONS:

CLINICIAN:_____

FUNCTIONAL COMMUNICATION RATING

Syracuse Voice Center
SUNY Health Science Center
Syracuse, New York

(appropriate for completion pre- and posttherapy)

Patient: _____   Date: _____

TO BE RATED BY PATIENT:

	Agree	Uncertain	Disagree
1. Before surgery my speech was easy to understand.	☐	☐	☐
2, My speech problem interferes with my job.	☐	☐	☐
3. My speech interferes with family relationships.	☐	☐	☐
4. My speech interferes with my social life.	☐	☐	☐
5. My speech requires a lot of effort.	☐	☐	☐
6. Speaking causes me pain or discomfort.	☐	☐	☐
7. I have to strain to talk.	☐	☐	☐
8. Some people have trouble understanding me.	☐	☐	☐
9. Most people have trouble understanding me.	☐	☐	☐
10. People seem bothered by my speech.	☐	☐	☐
11. My speech embarrasses me.	☐	☐	☐
12. I am annoyed when asked to repeat.	☐	☐	☐

TO BE RATED BY CLINICIAN: FCMVD Voice Disorder

Level 0   Unable to test.

Level 1   Vocal production is nonfunctional for communication.

Level 2   Vocal production is functional for brief episodes; most communicating must be done by nonvocal means.

Level 3   Vocal production is unreliable, although some voice communication may occur in limited contexts.

Level 4   Appropriate voice production is limited. Self-monitoring and self-correcting skills are inconsistent. Voice is distracting to most listeners.

Level 5   Appropriate voice production is consistent in most contexts. Self-correcting skills are used appropriately. Voice quality is distracting to some listeners.

Level 6   Voice production is appropriate in most situations, although minimal difficulty may occur.

Level 7   Voice production is normal for all speaking situations.

The following questions are only applicable posttherapy.

1. Patient has followed the therapy protocol with ☐ full compliance ☐ partial

compliance ☐ noncompliance

2. Patient's emotional status has interfered with therapy goals. ☐ agree

☐ uncertain ☐ disagree

3. Patient's physical status has interfered with therapy goals. ☐ agree

☐ uncertain ☐ disagree

4. Patient is comfortable using alaryngeal speech. ☐ agree ☐ uncertain ☐ disagree

5. Patient would be a good role model for others. ☐ agree ☐ uncertain ☐ disagree

---

APPENDIX

G

Some Useful and Interesting Websites

Title	*URL*
Academic Sites	
Archives of Otolaryngology— Head and Neck Surgery	www.ama-assn.org/public/journals/otol/ about.htm
CA: List of Issues	www.ca-journal.org/frames/front/issues_frame.
General Information	
CDC's TIPS: Tobacco Information and Prevention Source	www.cdc.gov/tobacco
LARYNX-C: The Larynx Cancer Online Support Group	tile.net/tile/listserv/larynxc
Cancer of the throat or larynx	www.healthanswers.com/database/ami/ converted/0010.42.html
Cancer Guide: Basic Information on Cancer	cancerguide.org/basic
David L. "Dutch" Helms' Home Page	members.aol.com/fantumtwo/index.htm
Facts on Cancer of the Larynx (InHealth)	www.inhealth.com/aboutc.htm

Title	URL
Healthtouch—Speaking After Laryngectomy	www.healthtouch.com/level1/leaflets/aslha/aslha051
National Cancer Institute	icicc.nci.nih.gov/clinpdq/pif/Laryngeal_cancer_Patient.html
Introduction to Alaryngeal Speech	www.ahs.uwo.ca/orcn/asha
Laryngeal cancer	www.meb.uni-bonn.de/cancernet/101519
Laryngeal Cancer (Virginia Voice Center)	www.voice-center.com/larynx_ca
Laryngeal Cancer Information	members.aol.com/fantumtwo/cancer1.htm
LARYNX-C: The Larynx Cancer Online Support	www.tile.net/tile/listserv/larynxc.html
MedicineNet Home Page	www.medicinenet.com/Index.asp?li=MNI
SEER Homepage	www-seer.ims.nci.nih.gov
Surgical-Prosthetic Voice Restoration Following Laryngectomy	www.odyssey.on.ca/~panda.prod/alaryng
The American Joint Committee on Cancer	www.facs.org/about_college/acsdept/cancer_dept/programs/ajcc/ajcc.
Laryngeal Carcinoma in situ	www.unsw.edu.au/clients/stgeorge/cis_glot.htm
American Cancer Society	www.cancer.org/frames.html

Companies

AddVox	www.stantonmagnetics.com/catalog/page16.
Bivona - Optivox	www.bivona.com/index.htm
InHealth	www.inhealth.com
Jack Kemp Enterprises	www.mcniffetc.com/jackkemp
LarynxLink, The Laryngectomee Shopping Mall	www.larynxlink.com
Lauder Home Page	www.voicestore.com
Provox	www.bedrijfsnet.nl/~wgrolman/provox.htm
Servox Electrolarynx	www.siemens-hearing.com/pprods/servox.html
UltraVoice	www.ultravoice.com
UMI (ProQuest Medical Library)	www.umi.com

Title	URL
Other Web Sites	
5pSP27 Tongue prostheses for articulation	Sound.media.mit.edu/AUDITORY/ asamtgs/asa94mit/5pSP/5pSP27
Cancer Sites: Oral Cancer	Www.salick.com/resource/siteo01
Detecting & Preventing Oral Cancer	Www.emerald-empire.com/zines/health/
Detecting Oral Cancer The Extraoral Examination	Www.tambcd.edu/oralexam/exam01.htm
Facts About Oral Cancers	Www.MedNews.net/dental/Bobier.html
	Www.mediconsult.com/noframes/general/ shareware/oral/contents.html
Healthtouch - Speech, Hearing & Learning Disabilities	Www.healthtouch.com/level1/leaflets/ 111717/111717.
Lip and oral cavity cancer	imsdd.meb.uni-bonn.de/cancernet/102840
	www.noah.cuny.edu/cancer/nci/cancernet/ 202840.html
	wellweb.com/INDEX/QORALCAN.HTM
	www.oralcancer.org
	www.catalog.com/dentist/orlcnr.html
Oral Cancer Professional Resources	www.oralcancer.org/profile.dir/educatio
SPOHNC (Support for People with Oral and Head and Neck Cancer)	www.spohnc.org

REFERENCES

Aguilar-Markulis, N. V. (1986). Reestablishing swallowing and speech after oral and pharyngeal surgery: A challenge for speech pathology and prosthetic dentistry. In W. Carl & K. Sako (Eds.), *Cancer and the oral cavity*. Chicago IL: Quintessence Publishing.

Allison, G. R., Rappaport, I., Salibian, A. H., McMicken, B., Shoup, J. E., Etchepare, T. L., & Krugman, M. E. (1987). Adaptive mechanisms of speech and swallowing after combined jaw and tongue reconstruction in long-term survivors. *American Journal of Surgery, 154,* 419–422.

American Cancer Society. (1990). *Cancer facts and figures*. Atlanta, GA.

American Cancer Society. (1996). Guidelines on diet, nutrition, and cancer prevention: reducing the risk of cancer with healthy food choices and physical activity. *CA— A Cancer Journal for Clinicians, 46,* 325–341.

American Joint Committee on Cancer. (1997). *Manual for staging of cancer* (5th ed.). Philadelphia: Lippincott-Raven.

American Speech-Language-Hearing Association. (1990). AIDS/HIV: Implications for speech-language pathologists and audiologists. *Asha, 32,* 46–48.

American Speech-Language-Hearing Association. (1992). Guidelines for evaluation and treatment for tracheoesophageal fistulization/puncture. *Asha, 34*(Suppl. 7), 17–21.

American Speech-Language-Hearing Association. (1992). Code of Ethics. *Asha, 34*(Suppl. 9), 1–2.

Aust, M. R., & McCaffrey, T. V. (1997). Early speech results with the Provox prosthesis after laryngectomy. *Archives of Otolaryngology—Head and Neck Surgery, 123*(9), 966–968.

Baggs, T., & Pine, S. (1983). Acoustic characteristics: Tracheoesophageal speech. *Journal of Communication Disorders, 16,* 299–307.

Blitzer, A., Baredes, S., Kutscher, A. H., Seeland, I. B., Barrett, V. W., & Mossman, K. L. (1985). *Rehabilitation of the head and neck cancer patient.* Springfield, IL: Charles. C. Thomas.

Blom, E. D., Singer, M. I., & Hamaker, R. C. (1986). A prospective study of tracheoesophageal speech. *Archives of Otolaryngology—Head and Neck Surgery, 112,* 440–447.

Brady, L. W., & Davis, L. W. (1988). Treatment of head and neck cancer by radiation therapy. *Seminars in Oncology, 15,* 29–38.

Brown, J. C., Zuydam, A. C., Jones, D. C., Rogers, S. N., & Vaughan, H.G. (1997). Functional outcome in soft palate reconstruction using a radial forearm free flap in conjunction with a superiorly based pharyngeal flap. *Head and Neck, 19,* 524–534.

Callanan, V., Gurr, P., Baldwin, D., White-Thompson, M., Beckinsale, J., & Bennett, J. (1995). Provox valve use for post-laryngectomy voice rehabilitation. *Journal of Laryngology and Otology, 109*(11), 1068–1071.

Carpenter, M. A. (1991). Clinical application of alaryngeal speech judgments. In S. J. Salmon & K. H. Mount (Eds.), *Alaryngeal speech rehabilitation: For clinicians by clinicians* (pp. 161–191). Austin, TX: Pro-Ed.

Centers for Disease Control. (1988). Morbidity and mortality weekly report. *Perspectives in Disease Prevention and Health Promotion, 37,* 377–388.

Chowdhury, C. R., McLean, N. R., Harrop-Griffiths, K., & Breach, N. M. (1988). The repair of defects in the head and neck region with the latissimus dorsi myocutaneous flap. *Journal of Laryngology and Otology, 102,* 1127–1132.

Christensen, J. M., & Weinberg, B. (1976). Vowel duration characteristics of esophageal speech. *Journal of Speech and Hearing Research, 19,* 678–689.

Clements, K. S., Rassekh, C. H., Seikaly, H., Hokanson, J. A., & Calhoun, K. H. (1997). Communication after laryngectomy. An assessment of patient satisfaction. *Archives of Otolaryngology—Head and Neck Surgery, 123*(5), 493–496.

Curtis, D. A., Plesh, O., Miller, A.J., Curtis, T. A., Sharma, A., Schweitzer, R., Hilsinger, R. L., Schour, L., & Singer, M. (1997). A comparison of masticatory function in patients with or without reconstruction of the mandible. *Head and Neck, 19*(4), 287–296.

Damste, P. H. (1958). *Oesophageal speech after laryngectomy.* Groningen, Netherlands: Haitsema.

Department of Veterans Affairs Laryngeal Cancer Study Group. (1991). Induction chemotheray plus radiation compared with surgery plus radiation in patients with advanced laryngeal cancer. *New England Journal of Medicine, 324,* 1685–1690.

Diedrich, W. M. (1991). Anatomy and physiology of esophageal speech. In S. J. Salmon & K. H. Mount (Eds.), *Alaryngeal speech rehabilitation: For clinicians by clinicians* (pp. 1–26). Austin TX: Pro-Ed.

Diedrich, W. M., & Youngstrom, K. A. (1966). *Alaryngeal speech.* Springfield IL: Charles C. Thomas.

Doyle, P. C., Danhauer, J. L., & Reed, C. G. (1988). Listeners' perceptions of consonants produced by esophageal and tracheoesophageal talkers. *Journal of Speech and Hearing Disorders, 53,* 400–407.

Drummond, S., Dancer, J., Krueger, K., & Spring, G. (1996). Perceptual and acoustical analysis of alaryngeal speech: Determinants of intelligibility. *Perceptual and Motor Skills, 83* (3 Pt. 1), 801–802.

Filter, M. D., & Hyman, M. (1975). Relationship of acoustic parameters and perceptual ratings of esophageal speech. *Perceptual and Motor Skills, 40*, 63–68.

Fitzpatrick, P. A., Gould, D., & Nichols, A. C. (1980). Self-administered intelligibility practice for esophageal speakers. *Journal of Communication Disorders, 13*, 341–346.

Flaitz, C. M., Nichols, C. M., & Hicks, M. J. (1995). An overview of the oral manifestations of AIDS-related Kaposi's sarcoma. *Compendium of Continuing Education in Dentistry, 16*(2), 136–138.

Franke, P. E. (1939). *Study of the rate of speech in words per minute and relation to judgments of rate.* Master's thesis, State University of Iowa, Iowa City.

Georgian, D. A., Logemann, J. A., & Fisher, H. B. (1982). Compensatory articulation patterns of a surgically treated oral cancer patient. *Journal of Speech and Hearing Disorders, 47*, 154–159.

Graham, S., Mettlin, C., Marshall, J., Priore, R., Rzepka, T., & Shedd, D. (1981). Dietary factors in the epidemiology of cancer of the larynx. *American Journal of Epidemiology, 113*, 675–680.

Greenspan, D., & Greenspan, J. S. (1996). HIV-related oral disease. *Lancet, 348*(9029), 729–733.

Greven, A. J., Meijer, M. F., & Tiwari, R. M. (1994). Articulation after total glossectomy: A clinical study of speech in six patients. *European Journal of Disorders of Communication, 29*(1), 85–93.

Grolman, W., Blom, E. D., Branson, R. D., Schouwenburg, P. F., & Hamaker, R. C. (1997). An efficiency comparison of four heat and moisture exchangers used in the laryngectomized patient. *Laryngoscope, 107*(6), 814–820.

Heaton, J. M., Sanderson, D., Dunsmore, I. R., & Parker, A. J. (1996). In vivo measurements of indwelling tracheo-oesophageal prostheses in alaryngeal speech. *Clinical Otolaryngology, 21*(4), 292–296.

Hilgers, F. J., & Schouwenburg, P. F. (1990). A new low-resistance, self-retaining prosthesis (Provox) for voice rehabilitation after total laryngectomy. *Laryngoscope, 100*, 1202–1207.

Hirano, M., & Bless, D. M. (1993). *Videostroboscopic examination of the larynx.* San Diego: Singular Publishing Group.

Hoops, H. R., & Curtis, J. F. (1971). Intelligibility of the esophageal speaker. *Archives of Otolaryngology, 93*, 300–303.

Hoops, H. R., & Noll, J. D. (1969). Relationship of selected acoustic variables to judgments of esophageal speech. *Journal of Communication Disorders, 2*, 1–13.

Horii, Y., & Weinberg, B. (1975). Intelligibility characteristics of superior esophageal speech presented under various levels of masking noise. *Journal of Speech and Hearing Research, 18*, 413–419.

Horowitz, A. M., Goodman, H. S., Yellowitz, J. A., & Nourjah, P. A. (1996). The need for health promotion in oral cancer prevention and early detection. *Journal of Public Health Dentistry, 56*(6), 319–330.

Hyman, M. (1955). An experimental study of artificial larynx and esophageal speech. *Journal of Speech and Hearing Disorders, 20*, 291–299.

Izdebski, K., Ross, J.C., & Roberts, W.L. (1987). An interim prosthesis for the glossectomy patient. *Journal of Prosthetic Dentistry, 57*, 609–611.

Kahrilas, P. J., Dodds, W. J., Dent, J., Wyman, J. B., Hogan, W. J., & Arndoffer, R. C. (1986). Upper esophageal sphincter function during belching. *Gastroenterology, 91*, 133–140.

Kaiser, T., & Spector, G. J. (1991). Tumors of the larynx and laryngopharynx. In J. J. Ballenger (Ed.), *Diseases of the nose, throat, ear, head, and neck* (pp. 682–746). Phildelphia: Lea & Febiger.

Kalb, M. B., & Carpenter, M. A. (1981). Individual speaker influence on relative intelligibility of esophageal and artificial larynx speech. *Journal of Speech and Hearing Disorders, 46*, 77-80.

Kawashima, T., Harii, K., Ono, I., Ebihara, S., & Yoshizumi, T. (1989). Intraoral and oropharyngeal reconstruction using a de-epithelialized forearm flap. *Head and Neck, 11*, 358–363.

Kelly, D. H., & Huff, C.L. (1980, November). *Esophageal voice utilizing a P-E segment pressure prosthesis.* A paper presented at the American Speech, Language and Hearing Association Meeting, Detroit MI.

Kesteloot, K., Nolis, I., Huygh, J., Delaere, P., & Feenstra, L. (1994). Costs and effects of tracheoesophageal speech compared with esophageal speech in laryngectomy patients. *Acta Oto-Rhino-Laryngologica Belgica, 48*(4), 387–394.

Landis, J. N., Murry, T., Bolden, S., & Wingo, P. A. (1998). Cancer statistics, 1998. *CA—A Cancer Journal for Clinicians, 48*, 6–29.

LaRiviere, C., Seilo, M. T., & Dimmick, K. C. (1975). Report on the speech intelligibility of a glossectomee: Perceptual and acoustic observations. *Folia Phoniatrica et Logopedica, 27*, 201–214.

Leder, S. B. (1994). Perceptual rankings of speech quality produced with one-way tracheostomy speaking valves. *Journal of Speech and Hearing Research, 37*(6), 1308–1312.

Leonard, R. J., & Gillis, R. (1982). Effects of a prosthetic tongue on vowel intelligibility and food management in a patient with total glossectomy. *Journal of Speech and Hearing Disorders, 47*, 25–30.

Leonard, R. J., & Gillis, R. (1983). Effects of a prosthetic tongue on vowel formants and isovowel lines in a patient with total glossectomy (An addendum to Leonard and Gillis, 1982). *Journal of Speech and Hearing Disorders, 48*, 423–426.

Leonard, R. J., & Gillis, R. (1990). Differential effects of speech prostheses in glossectomy patients. *Journal of Prosthetic Dentistry, 64*, 701–708.

Lewin, J. S., Baugh, R. F., & Baker, S. R. (1987). An objective method for prediction of tracheoesophageal speech production. *Journal of Speech and Hearing Disorders, 52*, 212–217.

Logemann, J. A. (1989). Speech and swallow rehabilitation for head and neck tumor patients. In E. N. S. Myers & J. Y. Suen (Eds.), *Cancer of the head and neck* (pp. 1021–1043). New York: Churchill Livingstone.

Logemann, J. A. (1994). Rehabilitation of oropharyngeal swallowing disorders. *Acta Oto-Rhino-Laryngologica Belgica, 48*(2), 207–215.

Logemann, J. A. (1998). *Evaluation and treatment of swallowing disorders* (2nd ed.). Austin, TX: Pro-Ed.

Loré, J. M. (1988). *An atlas of head and neck surgery* (3rd ed.). Philadelphia: W. B. Saunders.

Maniglia, A. J., Lundy, D. S., Casiano, R. R., & Swiontkowski, M. F. (1989). Speech restoration and complications of primary vs. secondary tracheoesophageal puncture following total laryngectomy. *Laryngoscope, 99*, 489–491.

Mashberg, A., & Samit, A. (1995). Early diagnosis of asymptomatic oral and oropharyngeal squamous cancers. *CA—A Cancer Journal for Clinicians, 45*(6), 328–351.

Matloub, H., Larson, D., Kuhn, J., Yousif, J., & Sanger, J. (1989). Lateral arm free flap in oral cavity reconstruction: A functional evaluation. *Head and Neck Surgery, 11,* 205–211.

McConnel, F. M. S., Adler, R. K., & Telchgraeber, J. F. (1986). Speech and swallowing function following surgery of the oral cavity. In E. N. Myers, I. Barofsky, & J. W. Yates (Eds.), *Rehabilitation and treatment of head and neck cancer.* (NIH Publication No. 86-2762). Bethesda MD: Government Printing Office.

McCroskey, R. L., & Mulligan, M. (1963). The relative intelligibility of esophageal speech and artificial-larynx speech. *Journal of Speech and Hearing Disorders, 29,* 37–41.

McEwan, J., Perry, A., Frosh, A. C., Cheeseman, A. D., McIvor, J., & Djazaeri, B. (1995, September 29). Surgical voice restoration: 15 years experience. In J. Algaba (Ed.), *Surgery and prosthetic voice restoration after total and subtotal laryngectomy.* Amsterdam, Netherlands: Elsevier.

Mendenhall, W. M., Parsons, J. T., Stringer, S.P., Cassisi, N. J., & Million, R. R. (1990). The role of radiation therapy in laryngeal cancer. *CA—A Cancer Journal for Clinicians, 40,* 150–165.

Merwin, G., Goldstein, L., & Rothman, H. (1985). A comparison of speech using artifical larynx and tracheoesophageal puncture with valve in the same speaker. *Laryngoscope, 95,* 730–734.

Michiwaki, Y., Ohno, K., Imai, S., Yamashita, Y., Suzuki, N., Yoshida, H., & Michi, K. (1990). Functional effects of intraoral reconstruction with a free radial forearm flap. *Journal of Craniomaxillofacial Surgery, 18,* 164–168.

Miralles, J. L., & Cervera, T. (1995). Voice intelligibility in patients who have undergone laryngectomies. *Journal of Speech and Hearing Research, 38*(3), 564–571.

Moon, J. D., & Weinberg, B. (1987). Aerodynamic and myoelastic contributions to tracheo-esophageal voice production. *Journal of Speech and Hearing Research, 30,* 387–395.

Morrish, E. C. E. (1984). Compensatory vowel articulation of the glossectomee: acoustic and videofluoroscopic evidence. *British Journal of Disorders of Communication, 19,* 125–134.

Morrish, E. C. E. (1988). Compensatory articulation in a subject with total glossectomy. *British Journal of Disorders of Communication, 23,* 13–22.

Myer, J. B., Jr., Knudson, R. C., & Myers, K. M. (1990). Light-cured interim palatal augmentation prosthesis: A clinical report. *Journal of Prosthetic Dentistry, 63,* 1–3.

Myers, E. N., Barofsky, I., & Yates, J. W. (1986). *Rehabilitation and treatment of head and neck cancer.* Bethesda, MD: Dept of Health and Human Services.

National Cancer Institute. (1988). *Oral cancers research report.* (NIH Publication No. 88-2876). Bethesda, MD: Government Printing Office.

Omori, K., Kojima, H., Nonomura, M., & Fukushima, H. (1994). Mechanism of tracheoesophageal shunt phonation. *Archives of Otolaryngology—Head and Neck Surgery, 120*(6), 648–652.

Ries, L. A. G., Kosch, P. C., Hankey, B. F., Miller, C. J., & Harras, A. (1997). *SEER Cancer Statistics Review, 1973–94* (NIH Publication No. 97-2789). Bethesda, MD: National Cancer Institute.

Robbins, R. T., Bowman, J. B., & Jacob, R. F. (1987). Postglossectomy deglutitory and articulatory rehabilitation with palatal augmentation prostheses. *Archives of Otolaryngology Head Neck Surgery, 113,* 1214–1218.

Robertson, M. S., Robinson, J. M., & Horsfall, R. M. (1987). A technique of tongue reconstruction following near-total glossectomy. *Journal of Laryngology and Otology, 101*, 260–265.

Ruhl, C. M., Gleich, L. L., & Gluckman, J. L. (1997). Survival, function, and quality of life after total glossectomy. *Laryngoscope, 107*(10), 1316–1321.

Salibian, A. H., Allison, G. R., Rappaport, I., Krugman, M. E., McMicken, B. L., & Etchapare, T. L. (1990). Total and subtotal glossectomy: Function after microvascular reconstruction. *Plastic and Reconstructive Surgery, 85*, 513–524.

Shipp, T. (1967). Frequency, duration, and perceptual measures in relation to judgments of alaryngeal speech acceptability. *Journal of Speech and Hearing Research, 10*, 417–427.

Skelly, M., Donaldson, R. C., Fust, R. S., & Townsend, D. L. (1972). Changes in phonatory aspects of glossectomee intelligibility through vocal parameter manipulation. *Journal of Speech and Hearing Disorders, 37*, 379–389.

Skelly, M., Spector, D., Donaldson, R., Brodeur, A., & Paletta, F. (1971). Compensatory physiologic phonetics for the glossectomee. *Journal of Speech and Hearing Disorders, 36*, 101.

Slavin, D. C., & Ferrand, C. T. (1995). Factor analysis of proficient esophageal speech: Toward a multidimensional model. *Journal of Speech and Hearing Research, 38*(6), 1224–1231.

Snidecor, J. C., & Curry, E. T. (1959). Temporal and pitch aspects of superior esophageal speech. *Annals of Otology Rhinology and Laryngology, 68*, 1–14.

Snidecor, J. C., & Isshiki, N. (1965). Air volume and airflow relationships of six male esophageal speakers. *Journal of Speech and Hearing Disorders, 30*, 205–216.

Spangler, J. G., & Salisbury, P. L. (1995). Smokeless tobacco: Epidemiology, health effects and cessation strategies. *American Family Physician, 52*(5), 1421–1430.

Spector, G. J., & Ogura, J. H. (1985). Tumors of the larynx and laryngopharynx. In J. J. Ballenger (Ed.), *Diseases of the nose, throat, ear, head, and neck* (pp. 549–602). Philadelphia: Lea & Febiger.

Sultan, M. R., & Coleman, J. J., III. (1989). Oncologic and functional consideration of total glossectomy. *American Journal of Surgery, 158*, 297–302.

Swisher, W. E. (1980). Oral pressures, vowel durations, and acceptability ratings of esophageal speakers. *Journal of Communication Disorders, 13*, 171–181.

Tardy-Mitzell, S., Andrews, M. L., & Bowman, S. A. (1985). Acceptability and intelligibility of tracheoesophageal speech. *Archives of Otolaryngology, 111*, 213–215.

Tiwari, R. M., Greven, A. J., Karim, A. B. M. F., & Snow, G. B. (1989). Total glossectomy: Reconstruction and rehabilitation. *Journal of Laryngology and Otology, 103*, 917–921.

Trudeau, M. D., & Qi, Y. Y. (1990). Acoustic characteristics of female tracheoesophageal speech. *Journal of Speech and Hearing Disorders, 55*, 244–250.

U.S. Department of Health and Human Services. (1986). *The health consequences of smoking: A public health service review, 1967–1985*. Washington DC: Government Printing Office.

Urken, M. L., Cheney, M. L., Sullivan, M. J., & Biller, H. F. (1995). *Atlas of regional and free flaps for head and neck reconstruction*. New York: Raven Press.

Urken, M. L., Weinberg, H., Vickery, C., Buchbinder, D., Lawson, W., & Biller, H. F. (1991). Oromandibular reconstruction using microvascular composite free flaps. *Archives of Otolaryngology—Head Neck Surgery, 117*, 733–744.

Watson, J. B., & Williams, S. E. (1987). Laryngectomees' and nonlaryngectomees' perceptions of three methods of alaryngeal voicing. *Journal of Communication Disorders, 20,* 295–304.

Weinberg, B., & Bennett, S. (1972). Selected acoustic characteristics of esophageal speech produced by female laryngectomees. *Journal of Speech and Hearing Research, 15,* 211–216.

Weinberg, B., & Moon, J. (1984). Aerodynamic properties of four tracheoesophageal puncture prostheses. *Archives of Otolaryngology—Head Neck Surgery, 110,* 673–675.

Weiss, M. H. (1993). Head and neck cancer and the quality of life. *Otolaryngology— Head and Neck Surgery, 108*(4), 311-312.

Weiss, M. S., & Basili, A. G. (1985). Electrolaryngeal speech produced by laryngectomized subjects: Perceptual characteristics. *Journal of Speech and Hearing Research, 28,* 294–300.

Weiss, M. S., & Yeni-Komshian, G. H. (1979). Acoustical and perceptual characteristics of speech produced with an electronic larynx. *Journal of Acoustical Society of America, 65,* 1298–1308.

Wells, M. D., Edwards, A. L., & Luce, E. A. (1995). Intraoral reconstructive techniques. *Clinics in Plastic Surgery, 22*(1), 91–108.

Williams, S. E., Scanio, T. S., & Ritterman, S. I. (1989). Temporal and perceptual characteristics of tracheoesophageal voice. *Laryngoscope, 99,* 846–850.

Woo, P., Colton, R. H., Casper, J. K., & Brewer, D. W. (1991). Diagnostic value of stroboscopic examination in hoarse patients. *Journal of Voice, 5,* 231–238.

Yang, P. C., Thomas, D. B., Daling, J. R., & Davis, S. (1989). Differences in the sex ratio of laryngeal cancer incidence rates by anatomic subsite. *Journal of Clinical Epidemiology, 42,* 755–758.

Zieske, L. A., Johnson, J. T., Myers, E. N., Schramm, V. L., & Wagner, R. (1988). Composite resection reconstruction: Split-thickness skin graft—a preferred option. *Otolaryngology—Head and Neck Surgery, 98,* 170–173.

INDEX